# SAM WOODS

# SAM WOODS
## AMERICAN HEALING

# Stan Rushworth

*Station Hill Press*
*A Talking Leaves Book*

A Talking Leaves Book published by Station Hill Literary Editions, a project of the Institute for Publishing Arts, Barrytown, New York 12507. Station Hill Literary Editions are supported in part by grants from the National Endowment for the Arts, a Federal Agency in Washington, D.C., and by the New York State Council on the Arts.

Edited by Peter Greenwood and George Quasha.

Text design by Susan Vaughan.

Cover photograph of Sam Woods by Megan J. Walch, Hobart, Tasmania.

Cover layout by Susan Vaughan and Guy C. Joy.

Distributed by the Talman Company, 150 Fifth Avenue, New York, New York 10011.

Library of Congress Cataloging-in-Publication Data
Rushworth, Stan, 1944-
    Sam Woods American Healing / Stan Rushworth
        p.   cm.

    ISBN 0-88268-122-2: $11.95
    1. Healing—Poetry.  2. Healers—Poetry.
I. Title
PS3568.U754S35   1993
814'.54—dc20                   92-81553
                                     CIP

Manufactured in the United States of America.

# Contents

Author's Note ix

Preface xi

The Resting Place 1

*Prayer for Keeping On* 4

Pravina's Talisman 5

*Prayer to Find It Everywhere* 10

Sorrow 11

Letter to Grandfather 15

*Prayer for the Earth* 20

Me and Pravina the Second Time 21

Animals 27

*Prayer to Hear My Fear* 32

Morning Coyote's Message 33

Thoughts for a Friend on the
   Medicine Trail 35

The Nature of Progression 39

At a Distance 44

Exploding 48

*Prayer for Sexuality* 51

Love and Understanding 52

*Traveler's Prayer* 56

Berlin Wall 57

*Prayer in Germany* 59

Workshops and The Butter Lady 60

| | |
|---|---|
| *Prayer to Find the Silence* | 73 |
| Silent Anger | 74 |
| *Life Prayer* | 76 |
| Motive | 78 |
| *Prayer to the Teutonic Gods* | 84 |
| Dilemmas | 85 |
| *Prayer for Dealing with Bullshit* | 90 |
| A Note on Healing | 91 |
| *Desperation Prayer* | 98 |
| *Prayer to Move Through Darkness* | 100 |
| Dreams | 101 |
| *Prayer to Where Bitterness May Lie Unattended* | 106 |
| Seizure | 107 |
| *Song Prayer* | 112 |
| Crystal Power | 113 |
| *Obligation Prayer* | 117 |
| Saturday Munich | 118 |
| *Prayer for Completion* | 119 |
| Meeting a Baby | 120 |
| *Home Prayer* | 123 |
| Loneliness | 124 |
| *Prayer to Reach You at a Distance* | 128 |
| The Vanishing Nature of Revelation | 129 |
| *Mountain Traveler's Prayer* | 134 |
| A Quick Beginning | 135 |

| | |
|---|---|
| *Prayer for Healing* | 138 |
| Concepts in Healing | 139 |
| *Sun Prayer* | 143 |
| Instant Healing | 144 |
| Something Big | 146 |
| What Do We Know About the Ancestors? | 148 |
| *Time Prayer* | 151 |
| Who's Safe Anymore? | 152 |
| *Prayer of Thanks* | 156 |
| American Beauty | 157 |
| *Prayer for Accidental Meetings* | 166 |
| Spirit Dance | 167 |
| Fear and Leaving | 170 |
| *For the Manner of Our Continuation* | 177 |

# Author's Note

Though I've run across Sam Woods for many years, I first really got to know him one night in the Intensive Care Unit of a local hospital. A friend of his had stopped breathing and lay on the border between living and dying, her body hooked up to life support systems. Sam lay on the floor and prayed for a long while, then got up and talked to her, though she was paralyzed and unconscious. The doctors had paralyzed all but her heart so her body wouldn't reject the tubes entering her from the machine that breathed for her. They had given her amnesiac drugs so she wouldn't wake up and panic, see the situation she was in, and suffer heart failure from the fear. Sam whispered into her ear, looking at all the equipment, telling her she was well taken care of. Then he lay back down on the floor for another long while, lying very still except for his lips, which moved almost constantly without sound. He did this over and over all night.

Before dawn the attending nurse told Sam in quiet tones that unless his friend's heart rate came down soon, they were going to lose her. Sam nodded, then lay back down on the floor again, but not for long. He rose quickly, then held his friend's wrist, touching her shoulder with his other hand. He stared at the digital heart monitor, and spoke softly, "Let my heart become hers." There was a brief pause, then a peace seemed to move through them both, and the monitor dropped from one twenty-eight to seventy-eight. Sam said "Thank you" very quietly, leaned down to kiss his silent friend, then lay back down to pray.

Since that time I've gotten to know Sam a lot better, and this book is his story, told his way. It's his way of moving through the world.

Stan Rushworth

# Preface

This book isn't about anything but what I see going on around here. I was going to write about love, and about healing, and how the two work together. I was going to write a book of prayer, because it's such a good way to get by, and it goes so far inside of you to get the good prayers, cleans you up from the inside out. Then a friend of mine said I should write about the Cherokee mind-body-spirit stuff, again around healing, and we talked for awhile about that 'til we both started laughing and decided none of it can be detailed down into any name or system. There's way too much of that stuff going on already, and once you call it something it all turns to dust anyway.

I had wanted to make something people could use to take care of each other with, something that would live inside of someone to say the best way to take care of yourself is to take care of somebody else, because I see everybody trying to love themselves so they can love someone else. "Got to love yourself first," they say, and I kind of shake my head as I walk away, because it seems to me that's the whole problem in the first place, this separation. And how can there be a 'first' in loving someone? I don't understand this stuff. Every time I see somebody concentrating on loving themselves I see the eyes closed, or glazed over with all the doors closed save one or two, and I can't figure out how to even reach them there's so damn many rules all over the place. I keep listening, and asking what's going on, but nothing real ever comes down past that point. They might sit there for a minute or an hour loving themselves, then they come back and the smile they bring with them is way out in left field, like from another planet. I keep not seeing much love there, but a whole lot of something else I can't define, and don't much care to, because it's so removed. It's hard to describe something so far away.

Now I promised myself I wasn't going to go on about loving, because I'm no expert in the matter, but I do know what I like, and I feel old enough now to say what I'm seeing. And I see a whole lot of shit that's polished up to look like gold or God, while it ain't nothing different than it ever was, and that's just lies, plain and simple. And I don't say this from any distance, but from inside the truth of my own lies, the ones I've lived, still live, and feel some kind of stupidity around. I'm not about to say I've arrived anywhere and have any secret or any kind of great revelation. Grace and The Fall keep on happening all the time, the way I see it, and there's little anyone can do to change that, as hard as we might try. It's like breathing, in and out, and it can't be grasped for long, no matter what kind of beatific face we might put on it. The guru finally gets jealous just like any other man, and the sage still farts at the wrong time. The genius won't get the punch line of every joke, and this is much to the common man's benefit, if we will only allow it to be so.

But we do like to worship ourselves in the face of the next person, regardless of how empty and tiresome it may become, to make a path to last us a lifetime. We build up ethics to avoid things, or to live only in certain things to the exclusion of others, and in this we build certain prisons, not only for ourselves, but for everyone around us.

And this is the crux of what I want to say, that we must look at the prisons we build for others, because we can't see ourselves that clearly, just by the nature of the beast. We can only get so far outside ourselves, and introspection too only goes so far, and the Yogi almost always comes out of the cave glad to have somebody to talk to, or just to play ball with. It always comes down to simple things, like sharing, smiling with a child, or holding the face in the sun. It's my belief that we can go straight to this without so much time apart. Modern life is already as much of a cave as we can handle.

It's already a monastic life we live, facing Zen Nothingness on the tube or in the newspapers or in a million seminars illuminating the darkness or taking us back into our mother's blood. I don't mean to belittle any of these things, as they are all valuable, but to say that the center of what we are searching for is all around us every day, if we would only stop and take a look.

So in that spirit, I am offering all the words you'll see in this book. It doesn't say anything different than what's been told a thousand times before. It's just another voice crying out, like someone hooting at a football game. It's me hollering at all of you, and at myself, sometimes speaking soft, sometimes frustrated, sometimes turned all inside myself in pain reaching out for some kind of connection. Other times everything's all laid out in front of me in peace, and these things are in here too. I just feel that it's my turn to say my piece, and I offer all this in friendship. I feel like we're at a party playing charades, and I'm just now standing up trying to say something by pointing here and there, making big eyes, slapping different parts of my body and hoping it somehow comes across this crazy gap between us all.

Sam Woods

# SAM WOODS

*In the first light of morning, may we remember*
*the magic. May the white sun explode through our eyes*
*on the name of our love. May we remember.*

*And in the evening, when darkness settles into our*
*bones, stars kindling the beginnings of dreams, may we*
*remember. May we always remember.*

# The Resting Place

Things have been happening. A woman comes from Tasmania, part white, part Aborigine, sometimes all Aborigine, fierce and docile all at once, sometimes all white, terrified and guilty all at once. In the night, my hands touch her belly and she sobs, and children roll out of her across rolling plains by a cold sea, their dark hair and wondering faces staring into the lives they will lead. I touch her hips and they become the parameters of her picture of herself, something huge, misshapen and ugly shrinking down into her reality. "I am not bigger than this," she thinks. Inside, there are the old ones waiting, laughing to her mind, her memory, her longing. Her body is waiting to live. She has been bedridden for three years. She sobs. She wails, and my hands rest on her womb quietly. I see darkness, shapes of mountains and stones, and I listen to her assistance, to the old ones, and to the living ones too, and we all beseech each other to be a soft part of this infusion, as it enters her from the belly, and from the knees, and from the shins, and from the hip-bones, moving

1

upward through her uterus and solar plexus and tortured heart, torn throat, face, into her dark shining eyes, and suddenly, like birds bursting into the sky she smiles across it all in soft abandon, and grief leaves far into the night, flying away in a desire to inhabit someone else, something else, another place. And she begins to know she can live. On the phone to Tasmania, she tells her friends that she is completely well.

One week later she has another body, with the same mind racing through it, wondering how to inhabit it. My hands rest on her shoulder, moving slowly, and terror raises its head, dead ones moaning, guilt, notions of lies, and lies themselves walking all across her breast, deep inside where she is transparent, and long voices peel her open from the bottom of her existence. It is horrible, and hot tears spread across her face onto my wrist, my forearms, cooling quickly in the night, burning my skin. Pale light curls her form below me, and I hear the old ones voicing their being, without understanding their words, only sounds from this moment that stretches in all directions without end, but with purpose, to give name to injustice, to blindness, to cruelty, to the death of a people, and a way of knowing.

We wait. Then my hand stops in the soft flesh above the hipbone. "There," she says, and her body breaths again, breaths out and sinks down into the earth and her face goes passive, nothing visible in her expression but waiting and relief. There is only the sound of breathing. Then she sighs and there is gentleness, and the smile I remember slowly fills her face, fills her mouth, fills her eyes, and spills into the three-quarter moon night, becomes the mist that holds the gum trees, and a sacred song washes all the past into what we live now. It lifts her upright by her lips, by her glowing eyes, her radiant hair, her soft belly as she sings and looks love into me from where she sees.

I walk into the night. For a moment we stare down the moonlit valley together, this a silent prayer. Luminosity is the nature of our being, and again the moment expands endlessly outward. I walk down the long wooden stairway to my cabin slowly and the sky folds a blanket of centuries around me. I lie within the confines of my heart and dream of nothing different than what I know. There is peace and great meaning everywhere, and something easy grows all over the face of the earth, while frogs sing to each other across the meadow.

## Prayer for Keeping On

*Let us find a way to keep it moving, to keep it alive and free, where it wants to be. Let us walk all the way through doubt consistently, to believe in what we have found in our beginnings. Let us know what is real, and let us pass it back and forth between our hands until we are gone from this earth, and even then, let us remain in this spirit, please.*

# Pravina's Talisman

Ahh my heart is full with your voice, so full with life. You sing of sadness and loss, and I see this, hear this echoing into my own cells, libraries of cells going endlessly into a blue universe, fluorescent. You came from the bottom of the world, but you are of this land; it is in your voice, in the rhythm and the drive. You have been me, and our hands have touched the wounds together, made the circles east and west, from where we came, to where we go. We have turned circles, backs toward one another across continents, come round to face each other again and opened our hands to the mother. We have sung, then given our skin to the ground to heal the tear in her body. We have watched the three-quarter moon and heard the wolves howl. We have stared long into the lizard's eye. We have listened to the magic resonate through centuries, and our parents look different eyes through the same faces, seeing this history. We stand with one foot in the water and one on land, our faces broken into halves that hold each other

5

tenderly, mending, piecing together the old and the new, carrying everything with us as we go.

By the lake's edge we stand silently; there have been many such cold nights. Your eyes extend in spheres around us, gentle, wary and sure. There are no questions. Voices laugh in the background and we smile at each other. Can it be hard? What can we see in this tonight? Every time must be different, and you have passed this sound to me of your questions, and your passion, where we have traveled into the blood to find a home, where we have met more friends than could ever be imagined, more beings willing to help in this time, this place so far in image from what their home was. Yet still, it is the same, your face in the moon, first white, then black, always shining of the same hue, and your scowl of protection, the warrior ready, and ready for the softness, the yielding as well. I nod to you. We are back here to pass the medicine again in honor and supplication. The gum trees stand guard over our witnessing, our prayer circle, and the mix of languages gives birth to common vision, a blending of sound like the owl and the frog. It is a time to give thanks, and to join the laughter of the ancestors.

Just what is it that we are to do? There is something speaking to me here on the edge of what I understand, something I see, have seen and most surely know, but the form is only now emerging. The solar plexus reaches out a hand of old magic and claws some sky into its grasp, holds it to the warm sun, watches it melt into a snow of knowing, a carrying of food for the hungry spirit to take on its way. Yes, I see how this is to be, how strength will be born and sustained with the wills of the old ones who stand with you. I see the shoulders sprouting long fingers that hold you between the stars, feet descending far below the surface of the earth, to where the soil is warm and flowing, curling between your bare toes, infusing you with gentle fire. Your knees send lines of light down into the trees, who hold you upright, make you pliable in the wind, fill you with the smells of their leaves, the colors of this spring. When you squat in the night, looking upward, your falling urine is liquid spine dipping into the earth, who fills you with herself, fills your organs, your bowels, your stomach, your lungs, with her richness, a soil of light. Your blood grows thick, full with all our bodies, the animals and us, the trees, autumn leaves and the moisture of yesterday's gentle rain. From your neck there is a radiance of circles, discs reaching outward to become clouds, fecund and delicate, rolling on a carpet of sound like chimes. Your face is made of rose petals to hold your eyes, and your ears are all the sounds that are made. There is no separation anywhere and you are protected by all who hear you, and by all you hear. Your hands are free, and your movement is buoyed by the surging of the stars, the pulsing and the dance that moves with you as though your lover, holding you in the tenderness and strength that comes from knowing, from seeing what it takes to live, allowing your will to cry into the center of the remnants of your obstinance, the last vestiges. Your rest comes into motion as an ancient hand strokes the fur of your wolf and smooths the feathers of your owl, dark fingers rich with sun and forests, open seas beside huge circular stones, eyes in the shapes of earths.

We here sing in the night of your coming, listen to your stories and see your world, what you see of ours, this same one. We bow our heads with no need to invite the silent ones; they are present, each an emissary for the other, even humor present in the midst of the obvious horrors. We sit in a dark night in silence to give you our talisman and our request from all the gods that be, the spirits who protect and guide us, all the kindly forces of us. We lay this bundle before you in which the message of this land may protect you and guide you as you travel easterly across her heart. We send this flesh with you for joining, and we open the boundaries that we may travel together wherever needed.

It has gone on too long to do otherwise, and this is what the smile says, what the eyes say, and what the rhythms keep delivering. Listen. I hear intense quiet, then the rumble of distant laughter, a chiding and a kind eye, a giving eye. Yes. What is it? There is a moment of technology in all these forests and vast landscapes, a glowing box of institutions holding all our words, the shells of forgotten people who insist on returning. They know what simply is, what must be, and they enter us with no struggle as we stride boldly into the center of our time. We are children in our favorite clothes, wearing the magic bandana, the hat that smells of grass and adventure, yet we are bound in choiceless abandon to the will of time and circumstance and history all stuck together into a brew of our own miraculous doing. We pass this gift along of knowing each other, trading sounds and sights across the boundaries of the body and the memory in ways we know and ways of mystery we can't even touch all at once. How can we not open our hands in awe and gratitude as the stones and words tumble all around us from a horn of plenty? How can we not become the world who so fills us? How can we not be the smiling warriors of the great medicine wheel? How can we not?

## Prayer to Find It Everywhere

*There's so much missing, so many places the magic goes awry, but let me find it everywhere, in cross-country restaurants, waitresses with an easy smile, in people at crosswalks and crossroads, everywhere, each day at least in little ways. Let me not focus on what can't be done, but on what's here, who's here trying, doing it, offering it freely, for their own desires. Let me find these people and spread their tale too, of how this came to be, of why it is, of what we must see and do. Let it fall easily, any way it can, before my open eyes. Let the simple reach me, and let me answer from the heart. Let me return each greeting in respect, always knowing how far we've come, and how much it takes to bring it all together, every time. Let me find it in the midday train whistle, and the distant barking dog. It's good from here, and keeps on going everywhere it needs to. Let this be.*

# Sorrow

Sorrow's train comes easily in the middle of the night, from everywhere, Indian children by the roadside staring with big tearless eyes, an old medicine man with his head tilted back toward the sky silently, hands open and pleading. Someone described me recently, young from a distance, older when close, wrinkles around the eyes talking a joy of living, and secrets beneath to use when needed to try to find the place. Always my face is the same to me, when it's a stone mask or an opening day of love; always it's thousands of years the same face, mine but not mine, owned by thousands, all my makers rolling through this heart that betrays my knowledge with change on top of change.

Everything comes to be on the surface for me, and I dance this way and that, call to the four directions, yet there is nothing I can do. I am twisted into the shapes of the world I live in, sometimes a gossamer cloud drifting across the day, and then I want to be this way forever, but the clouds gather and villages pray for rain to water their corn, and we fall to

11

the earth together, grow into tall corn, and are eaten by the same mouths from which we speak. Other days I crouch motionless beside my mother, a huge breathing rock, a cold stream rushing by, snow melting across the meadow as Spring blooms the first birds into the air. Still, I see the beginnings, and when the sun strikes my face the moss begins to grow. Cold dew drips down my cheeks.

I watch tears fall for no reason, because no reason is needed any more. There is no arm to grab when the spin begins, like when the rabbit runs for his life in the war of a moment, a dispassionate eye flying down through the air on a wind of talons. Yes, there is the love that does not cease, and the sorrow that visits like family, filling every room of the house, easy to see, easy to live with all day long, long into the night breathing after the fires have gone out and only stars light its shape, the sleeping profile against the earth.

What can I do but listen? Even when there are no voices I must listen for the wind, for meaning inside and outside, for something to come to me to say it's all right. There is an explosion every day, a shadow of earthquakes in my body, a moment in which I see my death and feel my life, reflected in a woman's story of her children who face death daily, born this way, with birth defects, she tells me. They weren't supposed to be alive today, she says, but they are, and she figures they were born to create a face of courage to give us. I listen to her tell their story, and I see them in her womb, and the photographs now with a cigarette and a can of beer, standing on a beach at the bottom of the world, a sparkling sea beyond stark mountains that made this flesh she speaks from. Mother and daughter blend like a horizon and the sky then, like sorrow and courage grow from each other, passing from hand to hand on days when needed. Oh Lord come down to us now and find us here. Find us waiting.

Every night I listen, and as I do I always see the same valleys filled with animals and lines of people walking single file, spread out from one another, walking one foot after another with their thoughts, with their pride inside, their feet swollen from cold. I lean back and watch, and I wonder if I will ever stop seeing them, if I will ever see only the dancers around the fire, their faces lifted in ecstasy. It's a thought I laugh at, because I know there is no denial in time, no running, no blindness that stays. There is only to fold my people to my breast where I find them, and to lay my own head on the warm earth alone, when there is no one near. As I walk through these night mountains my throat swells with feeling, and I know deliverance is at best temporary, divine and full with the nature of inspiration. The faces around the fire call to me, but I watch from the edges of the woods, from the edges of civilization, my face pale in the moonlight, my eyes reflecting the fire. I am quietly bursting, my flesh extending out through centuries. I am one long prayer, and my sorrow is long. It is the broken hand dangling over a still sea. It is the half-lidded eye that stares unmoving. It is the ear that hears all there is to hear, the imagination that does not rest until light fills the cavity of my brain. It is the inclination, the desire, and the magic that has come to greet me.

# Letter to Grandfather

Grandfather, when I stood silently in that cold room where you lay small and frail facing the high ceiling, you were not dead, though your skull was empty and your eyes were closed. There was a moment when I saw your life with me alive in the room, and in that moment your spirit entered me, and I swore to all the gods I knew that I would live the value that you gave me, that I would stay in the center of the world, that I would listen to the animals, that I would find myself in the land, Aina. And now it's many years later that I see what has been done between us in this life, as I begin to see my work, your work, my father's work, and I hear his words talking of you, and my mother's words talking of you, and grandmother's eyes still holding what was between you.

Now I remember your ways that I have been living all these years, and I begin to understand how I came to stand on the outside, and I cry for both of us this separation from the world. Everything begins to change for me again, and I see the cycles for you over the years I was with you. I remember bringing in the cattle and watching squirrels, seeing you smile. You were gentle. You told me about killing, and you saw me kill my first animal; you saw me witness life leave at my hands, suddenly, and we both cried inside then for that loss that would never change. I remember what you told me about the craziness of the world, and how it was going to hell, all of it, that no one understood anymore, and I watched you over the years as you went inside and got hard edges around your eyes. You hardly spoke with people, yet still the animals understood, your old horse, who seemed he'd live forever. I knew you'd die soon after he did. And I remember how you softened in the last years, looking to touch again what hadn't been for many many years, the affection and the kindness, your smile and gnarled hand resting gently on grandma's shoulder, your sadness deep, and your courage in all the pain.

Did you know what you taught me? Did you know how long it would take me to understand? How did you deal with how far we had come away from the truth, all of us? Couldn't you tell me what it would be like on the outside for so many years? You were so far away from the schools and churches and libraries that you couldn't even see the separation in any way to give words to me. You only told me about what was in front of you, like when you threw the preacher off the land and told me "Any time some son of a bitch tells you what happens after you die, means he's got his hands in your pocket now." We were walking, you stomping in anger back out to the cows, who stared at you unflinching, as though they knew the same things you knew. I just begin to see how you knew, and I have lived this way all my life. But now I begin to understand.

There were the inventions, and the things you made us in the shop, and the time you took to ride with us, to walk along the ditch bank pointing out things to see. And there was the day hunters from the other side of the river were landing slugs all around us on the hillside til you crossed the river and came up behind them with the old double barrel 12 gauge. Your eyes were cold that day, and you told me about the dead cattle, left to rot, shot for sport. Nothing should be shot for sport, you said, and you told me why, and what animals could be shot, and when they could be shot. And you got up every morning at a time I didn't even know existed, because when we would eat breakfast you'd be coming in from the field, with the sun still rising, hungry. You'd put seven different kinds of cereal in one bowl and load it down with everything you could find, fruit and cottage cheese and brown sugar, and we'd be disgusted while you just laughed. You never said anything, but it became a ritual we could count on, to enjoy the beginning of every day. You were kind then, strong and soft.

I begin to see something again that passed in our blood, that mixed with the people from England and Ireland, and when I see this in my life, in the people around me, and the places I go for sustenance and to weep, I see where you lived the ways I live. I see how you taught me this those early years, and I wonder what you knew it was called. You never gave anything a name, nor talked of concepts and ideas. You just said what was there. And when you didn't know, you were silent, sometimes shaking your head and walking off. I now understand this.

I am at another great crossroads, grandfather, and I ask your advice. You speak to me deeply now, in genetic voices, in pictures that are very clear, and that emanate from the world around me. I am in the center of the world, most every day, and it is very alive. The hawks are still circling, and I ask of you the strength to listen more deeply, and to let this way emerge through my eyes and through my heart, and through my hands. I ask for strength, and for patience, and for the quickness to see. When you lay dead before me and your spirit passed into me I made a promise that keeps growing, that means we can never be alone, either of us, though we walk long valleys in silence with no animals to be found. It must take the next step, for all of us, and I know that this will happen, because I see it in the eyes around me. Are you awakening too, and is it time again for us to walk together? Are we to be given another chance?

Oh grandfather, you are one in a long chain who brought me into this earth to see, and I am trying, and I am learning, and there is so much pain in the people that I feel. I look long into the sky and there are people in all the forests, running and wandering and sweating blind. It is a strange time, and yet the ways are all blending and a powerful magic fills the air. It is very old, and circles are coming around and around so fast it makes the head spin. You were right; it's getting crazier and crazier, and at the same time it gets easier and easier to find the love that sustains and nourishes, because it is here everywhere I look, and the searching turns into the sorting before my eyes, this from that, all of the same hue, all of this world, faces cracking away to reveal the eyes of children in a long ago sun. Oh grandfather can you hear me tonight? Won't you tell me once again what I can't remember and help me in this huge garden. The animals are all thirsty, and there is much work to be done.

## Prayer for the Earth

*Let us just see it, simply, enough to drink in Spring's radiance, the yellow scotch broom against green fields. Allow our eyes to reach into the morning like fingers into wet grass, our tears falling into April's rain. We've been too long away, and the need is huge, our desire unsteady in this time. Let the invisible wanting burst to the surface of our skin, where we may know this world who holds us so dearly even in the middle of our blindness, and in the beginnings of our awakening. Let us lie face down in her beauty, feeding her with our gratitude. She is waiting.*

# Me and Pravina
# the Second Time

The moon speaks quietly through mist, outlining the Eucalyptus against the night. There was another healing tonight, as we found the resting place again, in a pocket of warmth just above the top of the hip bone. It's always a searching, and various pains shoot through the imagination in this finding, looking like dark places, black and white, good and evil. Fears surface quick and ugly, terrifying, thoughts of never finding any kind of rest, but only miles and miles of pain followed by a horrifying early death. But we keep moving forward, looking for the balance, seeing points on the body, and in the mind as best we can, to hold on by, places where the earth might touch a bone, places a song might be born or remembered, wading through what grows to be expected. Shit. Just shit, but always valid shit. Shit from a hundred years, or from more recent childhoods, or just some lousy radio station sending shit out through the airways. There's no telling what it is, and it defies all systems so it's almost pointless to build an understanding around it, from my point of view. Seems like every time I think I understand it, it moves to another spot and has another reason. It shifts positions, like a dog finding his place to spend the night, kind of blindly wandering half asleep, groggy and comical.

Ten days after the first touch the body seems like another person's sometimes, especially if its been waiting for a long time and has already done all its own preparation. It fairly leaps into another structure, and I know clearly what they mean when they say every piece of tissue is different every seven years, or whatever it is. The holding is a habit passed from one cell to the next ad infinitum, until the person, in this case the whole person tired of hanging out in pain, decides to freak out and damn near die or make some kind of change.

I suppose I could be approaching this from a scientific viewpoint, but that language is just too cold for me sometimes, though I do enjoy it, all that talk about bio-this and bio-that. I mean I know it's all true, and I like the rhythms and the knowledge and the distance, the objectivity, seeing how we're all part of the scheme of things, cogs in a great wheel, genetic products, shapes in the night coalescing into forms predicted by what went before us. I like it. There's a comfort, like a priesthood, and I can't complain about it because it sure as hell knows how to cut body parts and make pills that knock out some nasty bugs it'd take near forever to battle otherwise. But there are some ailments that you can't touch without dipping into the mystery, and these ailments are the ones of the soul. These are the ones that touch the environment, the pillaging of the heart, the land, the time, missteps over the edge of balance, when the body screams out from here, there and everywhere for no apparent reason, nothing that can be measured. I've seen more than one person come a hair's breadth from dying out of this.

It's here where we can help one another, and it doesn't take anything but an inquiring mind, a little sense of caring, and a lot of love. When I say love I mean the kind we all have for life, basic stuff. It's a matter of joining, which is what we're all searching for anyway. It's just that most of the time we're looking for money around this meeting, or sex, or obligations of I love you so you got to love me; this kind of stuff, and that won't make it where I'm talking about. It's got to be something else. You see, it's a listening, and that takes patience, because sometimes when you get in there, inside someone's body, all the demons in the world seem to be scratching at the door to get in, or to get out; it's all the same thing because the body starts writhing around and the breath stops and then the body gets stiff all over, which is probably what was already happening in one spot anyway, and fear sets in like a cold winter storm you just got to wait out. You just got to stay warm, keep stoking the fire, and pay no mind to the wind that's screaming around the corners of the house like a banshee. You got to bang a little on the body here and there, in opposite places, to let it know it's still on earth and nobody's taken it away into some dungeon. You got to tap on the shoulder, on the breast bone, to let the body hear itself awake. It'll do it on its own eventually; you just have to remind it that we're still on planet earth. Sometimes it's a matter of just holding a hand or an arm, or listening, or saying something that makes some kind of sense. Of course, nothing really makes too much sense then anyway, so there's always a quality of the unreal you have to cope with. This soon passes, thank God.

Then it gets real good, after the body begins to trust itself, and your hands, your humor, your having been there your own self maybe, in some way being able to know that together. This starts the breathing again, and when this happens is when the best part is, and when the real magic begins to work. It's like calling someone out in the night, and after a long hollering you finally hear them hollering back, and pretty soon they come trotting into the meadow all bathed in the light of the full moon. The breath begins to sigh, and all the pleasure wakes up, and memory isn't so bad anymore, and color comes back into being in the mind, and the demons do their strange alchemy of becoming gods of one sort or another, or at least allies. You can almost see the energy moving then, and sometimes you really can see it, clear as a bell, in the body, and in the eyes of course, glistening in the half-light, and this means the door is open. This is good, because here the body begins to help you and itself at the same time. It caresses your caress, welcomes touch like a thirsty sailor, and fairly blossoms second by second. Here is where the joy is begun.

The most important thing is to let it keep changing. You can't take any credit for anything that's happening here, that's for certain, and you can't forget that the "demons" banish themselves out of getting overtired with themselves. Just because they leave doesn't mean you've done anything the body doesn't already want to do on its own. It just needed a little jump start; that's all. And when it gets going is where delicacy really comes in handy, because it gets subtle before you know it. You have to follow real closely and keep your prayers straight. You have to keep them straight because here you and the other one aren't much different on the inside. In a way that's working before your eyes, you've become close, real close, so close you're almost the same person, and I suppose if you were really going to look at this, you could say you are the same people. It's a metaphor, and it's real, both.

But it's late, and I'm tired from a long day, so I won't go on about all this, but to say that when she started singing sacred songs again under this moon, looking into my eyes, I felt the blessing we'd just shared together and I wanted to live a thousand years so I could go on doing the same thing when the need was there. Only problem is the need is everywhere, so much you can't do it all or you'd never eat or sleep. Tonight was grand, though, because I'd been listening to it all week long, and knew what I wanted to see. I just didn't know exactly how to get there, and it took both of us to build that. It's like everything else; you got to give it the respect it deserves, no matter how you talk about it. It's a good thing, and needs to get passed on. Each of us has got the way suited best to ourselves, and it's in the wanting that it all gets born.

# Animals

The animals are the guardians. They are keeping the different parts of us alive. Without them we have no spirit, and we are only mind alone somewhere drifting without a home. The hawk is our sky, and the ground squirrel our feet. The coon is our cunning and the coyote the mischievous nature of our evolving soul. It's good to remember this, and to think of skunks and possums and fish and all creatures with strange faces and habits as our guardians.

I have met a group of dolphins on a number of occasions, in the middle of a vast, deep, beautiful bay. And I have heard about other dolphins, who spend time with children who cannot speak, who wish not to speak perhaps, or who are afraid to speak for fear of saying what they see. No one really knows why they don't speak, but it's seen that after these children are in the water with dolphins they speak very clearly, and they begin to inhabit their bodies in a new, more complete way. Perhaps the problems can be understood in terms of the nervous system, electrical charges not meeting, systems not coming full circle, energy damned up in the child somewhere somehow. But when the dolphins spend time pulling the children across the lagoon, connections are made and the children begin to learn, begin to speak, perhaps begin to see happiness in another light, as something that can fit here.

The dolphins that I met are grandfathers. We swim to the middle of the bay and wait for them, looking down into clear blue water, making shadows on the opacity with our bodies, long shafts of light reaching down from the sun to hold our shadows against the deep that can't be seen. They come when it's silent, and we are waiting. They come straight on, circling us, watching us from below, making direct passes through us, looking sideways, drifting with us, playing with us, imparting things we don't exactly know about. There is a change. People who are frightened stop being frightened, or they become so frightened that the fear runs up through their bodies like a dervish, twisting itself into grotesque shapes, an exit from normality into movement, but always with a good outcome. People are healed, plain and simple, and they begin to know love in another way.

There are aberrations here too, of people ingesting dolphins as world leaders, space creatures and surrogate lovers, but even in this there appears to be little harm but for some stasis tinged with outrageous drama, dreams implanted on this earthly reality.

More and more it seems that dreams can be a key. A dolphin held me in a dream once, then she died, and I sat crouched in the crevice of a huge rock, the sea spray on a violent day cast around me full of kelp and bitter salt smells, watching her funeral on the beach below. She was lying at the water's edge, people standing in a circle around her, looking down at her where she lay in a white cloth, flowers all over her body. I climbed down to hold her in my arms, kneeling in rough sand, rocks and broken shells, the waves hissing on the rocks behind me, reaching and withdrawing quickly like a threat. As I held her she became a woman and she opened her eyes to look into mine. She told me she was a woman on the land, and a dolphin in the sea, and then she closed her eyes and died again. Watching her become the dolphin again seemed to complete some kind of cycle for me that I couldn't name, and I knew she would be back. I awoke remembering another dream, one that was even present in my memory as I sat on the rock above her funeral.

In the other dream I was holding the prenatal form of a Tibetan child, watching him reach an age where he fell ill, folded in upon himself and died, rolling back then into decomposition and shapes of color, clear into a tumbling small mass of energy in my palm. His father, a Holy Man, watched with me, and when we looked at each other we knew that he and I and the child were keeping each other alive. Together we stared into the colors pulsing in my hand and the child's eyes formed to stare back at us, then his body began to follow his desire to live and he became a child in the womb, was born, and grew to the age where he died again. Inside of me these two dreams blended to become the same dream.

Now there is a real woman in my waking life who forms the dream again in another way. She becomes a cat guarding the temple around my heart, preventing intruders from entering the deepest reaches of me to draw my life from me, like the temple cats of ancient Egypt. In this I am given the freedom to live, and my strength then goes to her in balance, and I am the contented dog stretched on the dirt in hot sun. I am also the owl in the late night protecting her spirit from harm. I am the eyes that travel across great distances to give her sight, as she is the claw that opens my heart to the world again, my blood the rain that feeds the trees. We are the red-tailed hawks circling the meadow, watching the sheep and geese. She is the hummingbird that brings the healing, the fast heart beating, blurred wings on an emerald bosom. I am the fish breathing water in the middle of a night sky.

This is about the nature of allies, and there is gain here, and a furthering of the bond that heals. It is apparent that we are all here together in this whirling, looking for something to hold onto.

When I am in the woods or in the city, the animals are there to talk with, to find the ground for me again, and they know this. I can see it in their eyes. I look carefully, slowly, and their compassion overwhelms me. It picks me up and carries me across a day suddenly as though it is my whole life, and I see their place, and their frailty, their love, and the docility with which they approach their lives and deaths.

I close my eyes to listen, and I hear a red-winged blackbird call from long ago, in a field of alfalfa with a hundred of his brothers and sisters. He is calling through me, and I remember another of his kind who sits in a more recent memory, beside a pond in the hills above the city, at dusk in a stand of rushes, calling out the coming of the night. He sings with a thousand other birds, all singing together. They form a symphony that lasts as long as the sunset makes evening purple against winter branches, and when I walk back home, found in my proper place, frogs sing long about evening coming, and I must listen.

I must listen, because without them I am lost. Without their song the night will not come.

## Prayer to Hear My Fear

*I must listen to these voices. Wolf, protect me. Clean my wounds with your soft tongue. Owl, be my eyes in darkness. Illuminate my enemies. Soft wind, carry me gently from harm, to where my fear speaks in thunder, and I can see the way clear. Gather round me now and take me to where I belong. I am listening to you.*

# Morning Coyote's Message

There is a meadow in the desert, below a high peak, with red wild flowers in the foreground, lit by a sunrise that emerges from the folds of a distant thunderhead. There is a warm morning wind, and two coyotes pad across the plain below, their coats glistening in the first rays. It's easy to smile here, after a long evening of watching stars dance across the sky, liquid blue satellites moving like mercury through the heavens, this followed by dreams that emerge from love and a deep sense of fitness, taking hope into cupped palms and drinking freely around a small fire. And before that a plain meal eaten out of one pan, steaming in the evening, and before that a long day of hills and dusty paths, wildflowers midday, lizards staring from antiquity; it goes off into the past easily, like a shooting star.

It is easy to quickly fall into the morning coyotes, into their eyes, watching mice tracks etched by the sun's low angle, shadowed beneath moist gray-green plants, everything trembling in the morning desert way, everything beginning. We fall into the heart between their shoulder blades, deep down feeling the rhythm of the trot, soft like skating over the earth, skimming the giving soil, leaving almost no track at all, silent like an easy breeze. The smells fill the lungs and brain to make the eyes glisten. Inside, voices speak clearly.

"We turn toward the bluff, sensing something, and see two people standing high above us, their minds reaching toward us, gathering us into them, and we smile inside to see this intention. It is very good, clear and factual, simple in the heart, easy to see and to know, without fear. It is very good. They are building a memory for themselves and for us. We part from each other, turn a wide circle and come together again, and in this way etch our style into their day, all of us living together then for as long as we will breathe. They might wonder how we spoke to them in this manner, marveling to their friends about this morning, but deep inside they know our way, this way of the coyote."

# Thoughts for a Friend on the Medicine Trail

The Medicine Trail is a manner of approach, an attitude, like a color of dawn, something that reaches out to touch things any way that it can, unformed, created only by the desire to connect. Beneath all meetings there is the form given to us by time, by our forefathers. The patterns of the past reach out into the future both tenderly and boldly, reaching through our living bodies where we stand in this moment. This is the spirit of the Medicine Trail, that we are in the center of this movement, and that it is huge, grander than we can conceive. We must be buoyed by this, finally, and given great gifts when we approach in this manner of supplication. In this light our knowledge is a memory, not something we create. What we learn is huge, yet a shadow of the wind, the vanishing image of who leads us.

It is this, that when we are in a situation where suffering is prevented from changing into something else, that we are unafraid to listen, to understand, to hold ourselves in the center of this whirling and spin our own dancing circle. We don't know what will be given with this movement, but we know that change will occur, and that we will be watched, held and protected. We ask that the will of the land and animals be heard. We ask that the ancestors provide for us, knowing their presence. We listen. There are many gods present. We cannot tell them what must be.

It is this, that when the pain rises all around us a huge demon daring against the sun, crushing the spirit of our loving, of the loving in our people, we curl into a ball of prayer, of listening, of asking, of smallness. We take the power into the pit of our stomachs and begin to build warriors and gardens and promises and possibilities. We let the mind encompass every direction this might go, and hold true to our desire, knowing that this has weight in what might become to be. We look into the eyes to see what is there, knowing that in this vision there will be movement. We cannot know where we must go. It is much bigger than this.

It is that we have no choice. There is no doctrine, no teaching but some experiences passed on, maybe some herbs, or some questions, some things we might want together as a people, hopes against inevitabilities of the darker sides. When we see a child cry for no reason but for lack of a sense of place, what choice do we have but to listen? When someone's eyes spill over into our day in a great wash of confusion or sorrow, what can we do but listen? Can we turn our backs? And if we do, where can we go to avoid all these faces?

Listening in the middle of the night, what is there? Is the silence filled with the next steps for us, for her, the one who wept today at the loss of her family? Do the ghosts of those torn from this life before they were ready to go ask anything of us? What is our obligation to them? Listening in the world between sleep and dream, who is there? Do they provide us with something we carry into our day? Do they teach us strength? Do they frighten us into ourselves? Who is there?

And in the moments of the day when we do not know where we are, where we are going, or even who we are, in those tiny precious moments of delivery from being, who is there, and how long have they been listening? What is the deep cry that comes from the place we have not been inside?

There are many choices, until there is nothing left to chose from, and then this way of the Medicine Trail emerges like a great wealth. Tears may line its path, with little to be done to change this, and it may seldom fit any expectation, but it will always be. Even when the great darkness encompasses, this trail will always be. This is not our doing, but is the field in which we move.

I close my eyes to pray and listen. A woman sings from somewhere in the past, a rising and falling rhythm, her voice walking an invisible breeze. Tomorrow she will be held, and her eyes will fill with history. It can be heard in her song. She was born for this, and as she opens her hands to her life a softness rolls down her cheeks silently. She does not even feel the water, as voices fill her from the inside. All around her medicine falls from the sky, rises up from the rich earth, and blazes at her from a hundred fires, some burning in the eyes, others in the sky and on the ground. She will nurse the world as she sleeps. All around her the medicine burns, cools, rises into smoke, into clouds, into the softness in the dog's eye, into the morning bird's first call.

This way is the Medicine Trail. It is the place between the worlds from which we came and the worlds we will pass into. It is the alchemical brew of healing, the poultice made to cure the wound that opened when we were taken from the bosom of our maker. It is here, and nowhere else, and it will be this way for a long long time.

# The Nature of Progression

There's a gyroscope inside the body, whose electro-magnetic fingers reach out to touch the facets we call spirit, mind, and emotion. It builds a progression that's always seeking to occur, always moving, always bringing us to balance, despite our confusion, our camouflage, our sabotage. The aberrations from this are at best temporary, in a sense; even if they should last a lifetime, there is still a progression occurring in a part of the being that is saving us for knowing life in some profound and meaningful way. This gyroscope brings us only what we can handle most of the time, and when too much comes, there is still a compensation in areas that are unknown to us.

One minute I see someone sad on the stairways, surrounded by ivy and spring blossoms, and minutes later, she is smiling, seeing where she is, still knowing little or nothing, not knowing the reason for previously being unhappy, or whatever state that is we hate to be in because it's stopped, a trap, a leg iron, a cold place, a squinting in the eyes trying to see beyond the walls that keep coming up. If it's stasis that's so appalling and so prevalent, what is it that allows us movement?

This is a difficult subject to deal with, and requires equal doses of science and art. Big words.

I see progressions that continue to buoy me and to amaze me, and I wish to express an essential nature in these things, something that fills me with hope. There is a mechanism inherent in the body, as in the manner of a hawk who hunts for the weak of a species, keeping the strong breeding the strong. In this way he is part of creating a stronger and stronger world. There is no arrogance in him and he does not scorn the weak rabbit he eats; he knows his place in the scheme of things. It's seen in his eyes, and the human body has this same quality, inclination, and ability.

What I see is a deep tendency toward balance, and a source of this tendency that is beyond what we know or understand. It's always on the other side of our knowledge, a constant, an unknown, and it's both deified, held in check through this deification, and feared as much as anything can be feared. It's a tendency that is a great deal of things, all natural progressions of any world we might inhabit, any thought taken to its terrible or wonderful conclusion, and once arrived at, could be something magnified a thousand fold beyond our furthest expectations. It's like counting stars. I just want to acknowledge its presence, really, because definitions of it can only be temporary. Yet there are characteristics, styles, and manners in it that are always the same. It keeps going to the next level, making one feel larger or smaller, something different, yet somehow the same, and altogether familiar, though brand new. Paradoxes always wed in one form or another in this tendency, and allow greater amounts of juice to flow through the whole system, and it seems the more one invites this occurrence, the more is gotten from it. The main halting point in it seems to be a kind of greed, and is only found when the ear stops listening to all the voices concerned, all the myriad voices concerned, the ones speaking from everywhere at once, in dreams and living people, lovers and friends, politicians and priests, old radio stations still blasting away in childhood.

Everything seems to come with us everywhere no matter how hard we try to leave it behind. And everyone has all of it; it can be seen in droves of forms, heard in choruses of voices, and it's all alive all the time, nothing dying, nothing gone, though we might wish so at times and know then that if wishes were horses, beggars would ride.

Beneath it all there's a softness, a quiet humming, a center that is undeniable, connected to the middle of the earth and strung by strands of light measured and quantified by scientists, cool men with wild eyes and insatiable thirsts for knowledge. These strands of life make us the center between east and west, north and south, connect us with earth-made invisible twine to the exact middle of where we are, no questions asked. And in this connection of wires and sculptures and pulsations of twenty-first century lights and sounds, there is a path running all the way back in time to the beginning. It goes clear to the earth's core for its substance, for its fire, and for its steady burning.

There are a thousand ways to see it, many mystical notions, religious and scientific notions, yet its active presence is incalculable in value in a way that will not be captured. It deserves to be honored in a form that allows us to touch it in respect, to join it on its terms, believing if not in ourselves, then in the earth, in the joining, in the blending of the elements that compose us, and believing in the fact that this composition has occurred. The reasons why this has happened are personal, beyond generalization, but that it has occurred and that we are in the middle of it is a wonderfully undeniable fact every word attempts to describe.

All these words tumble in the center of what I see and try to say, so that we might come to our smile more quickly, or that we might join another person in gloom to boost the process into seeing flowers once again at one's feet, and thereby most certainly make the world better. It's just that it's natural, is what I'm trying to say, that the face of progression in all significant areas of personal and social evolution is consistent, has cyclic characteristics, many faces in the night, though it's powerfully ugly at times, yet the movement keeps on, and the urge keeps pure. The processes of listening and searching work well with this tendency, yet these in themselves are not answers to the breakdowns, the times when nothing is manageable, and you just want to go home even when you don't know where home is. There is no permanent handle, yet all of this is something we know, and perhaps what I seek to do is to say yes to this, and little more, yes to the fact that there is a quality of progression that is without question occurring which will be heard, which will not take no for an answer, insisting upon its own existence. That this lives within the body, within the person turning circles in the midst of mirages and centuries, is a great gift, and that there is no getting away from this, and that in the acceptance of this there is an endless capacity for anything, well, I don't even know what to say, but that this is very good.

# At a Distance

My love lives a day and half away by airplane, clear around the world. She comes to see me, and I go to see her, but we have chunks of time when we can't see each other, times when I wake up alone in the morning with an ache in my body all around where she should be, warm up against me. But we can't have this all the time, so I have to put another gear into motion, one that does the best it can to cover great distances and times. Like with everything else these days, this goes everywhere at once, into loving, and into healing on another level.

One of my elders gets sick sometimes, and when she does, I feel it. I see her body in my mind, with bright or dull light emanating from it, depending on how she's doing. It isn't specific at first, and it isn't the same every time, but there's always something to grab onto.

The first time I felt it strong I was in Hawaii, standing on a knoll looking out over the sea. I kept thinking her name, over and over, and so I sat down to feel what was going on, and that's when I began to see her. She had told me once that she used her own imagination as a backdrop for another person's psyche, and it made sense to me when I saw her that day in my mind. The thoughts were stronger than usual, and the images more captivating. There was a white fire struggling to get out of her chest, pulsating like a breath. I aimed my eyes into the center of this and it began to change. It never ceases to amaze me how much looking at something changes it, both in my own mind and in the situation that seems like it ought to have something active done to change it. Just looking at it does a lot, every time.

My friend's image kept coming back to me for a couple of weeks, and so I called her, and we had a good talk. She had been sick, and could feel me feeling her. Later, when I got back home, I worked on her body and even more changes started happening. I began seeing her a lot in my mind, and when I would, I'd just sit and concentrate on her, sending the best wishes I could. I called on Christ because I knew she felt close to him, that he was a strong presence in her life. She called me on the phone, laughing, and said "Are you working on me from a distance, you rascal?" She has a full and beautiful laugh, and she told me the effects of the work, so we had a corroboration between us that helped to further the bond and the effect.

45

Now I do this all the time, knowing that it somehow gets out into the pool friends can draw from. I worked on another person in the islands, with a bio-physicist there watching, and he and I talked a long time about how electro-magnetic energy moves through space and time. I came away feeling that prayer could be talked about in these terms, if the attitude stayed right, and he said all this fit perfectly with what he was learning in his field.

The only problem I have with quantifying these things is that we can lose sight of the source easily, and when a machine is built that approximates what the human will conjures in its desire to live coupled with another human will, then it's easy to say we understand. It's then that the owning of things can begin, and the mystery steps a bit further away, and when the mystery withdraws we're at the beginning of trouble. We think we've invented something, so we build a form to play with, in a fine desire for what we might provide mankind, and the next thing we know we've got another atom bomb. These propensities of the human being separated from nature frighten me.

But although we may be better off not knowing these things, we must move in the direction we figure is forward. My kids and I always sent love to each other through Orion, using him as a protector and general repository for anything we might need when apart. I've spent countless nights looking into his march across the sky, feeling them feeling me. It never seemed important that the timing was exactly synchronized, and the use of a constellation as a connector felt safe, and very permanent.

What I see is that everything I do enters the world somewhere, no matter what it is. Everything I desire or feel about someone goes somewhere, if only in a big circle back into myself. The incredible beauty of it is that the more I see this happen, the more it can happen, and sometimes it's so visceral I can touch it. I begin to know how to fit into places I never could before, and I get messages across to people without knowing them that well, or them understanding me. In this, my world becomes a smaller place geographically, and a much huger place philosophically. The philosophy becomes a living reality. The unity of things becomes a cause-way to ride on most anytime, a magic carpet I can touch the world through, thank God. In some ways this is all rudimentary, and in some ways not at all. In some ways it's on the furthest edges of what I could've ever hoped to know and live, and in others it's something that began the moment I was born, simply, without any choice in the matter.

# Exploding

A couple of years ago I told myself I felt as though I was about to explode, and now I'm feeling I already have. I hear the wind whistling by my ears, and I can't stop, even if I wanted to. It's a frightening prospect to consider, because I don't know what the explosion has begun, except that it's dropped me into this world in a different way, a composite of all my experiences looking different to me. Like right now, when I think about all this on a dark evening, I feel queasy in my stomach, like I'm going somewhere I've never been before, wondering if I'll be able to handle it. I want to address it, but feel it's something else now, something completely new to me.

The explosion used to be around the way I might hold a nipple between my lips, though even that had a certain reserve about it too often, and now everything melts together, holding my love close on an evening. It doesn't matter whether I'm inside of her in passion, or holding her back against my belly, warm into the soul. The explosion is here, everywhere. I feel like crying just to say it, as though I might die soon and already miss living.

It's like this. I touch her and breathe. I wait. What does she say? I listen deeply. We are finding something new to us, seeing how old our desire is. I need her here in this way, and I can't hold on too tight or she'll disappear, yet it is complete between us. Here my throat becomes something too full with itself to move, but it wants to badly, wants to sing like an angel, but it can't, so the feeling flies upward into the mind, where it looks for understanding, for pictures of the past and future, of where we'll go, but even there satisfaction is elusive. So it drops down into my hands where they slowly wander over her beauty, her upper arm, smooth and perfect, her breasts and sides, her stomach. I am searching, and her eyes gaze into mine with that expression that looks like sky or water, like a questioning and a knowing at the same time.

I am changing, waiting, moving body parts, listening to something coming apart inside of me, something that moves inwardly from my hands where they touch her, like splendor traveling into me up through my arms, through my veins, deep into my chest, looking for a place to become something huge, like a star reaching around itself into space, looking for a place to expand, or like a pregnant animal looking for a place to nest. Somewhere between these two things her love moves me steadily, here where I am mortal, and there, where the source of my life lies smiling at me. Sometimes she asks about my gratitude, about where it comes from, and about how I could so continually surrender to the incredible beauty of her letting down her hair, then tossing it all around her shoulders. It isn't the sensuality of this moment, though that in itself is enormous, but it's the way this connects to my whole life that matters, that explodes me into realization of her immediate presence. I can love her right now as fully as I can breathe, and as effectively. When I have my hand resting fully on the warmth of her sex, it becomes my eyes, seeing her, my nose, smelling her, my mouth, tasting her, and it tells the whole of me that I am in the right place, that this quality of diffusion, of expansion, and of explosion is a crossing over of all the senses and qualities of life into one great experience.

How could I ever want to exist separately from anything again after this? I pray from the bottom of my being that this will never lessen, no matter what form it may want to take, and that every part of living that touches me will be the manner in which I am held together. She provides both the explosion and the coming together, and this is why I am so grateful. She is my companion in this raging wind, everywhere we are taken.

# Prayer for Sexuality

*Easy, reaching down, allowing, falling into place, moving like fire along a dry branch, illuminating the darkness. Let it be this. And like rain touching grass, falling against the green and flowing down into the earth to disappear. And like sun warming the cat's fur. Let it be these things. May it take me into knowing everything each time complete, holding life in my hands. I ask for this to feed me now, for the rest of my life, to feed me fitness each time, release, and steady gentle strength. Then may the nature of it reach out to touch the world steadily, gently and quietly. May it be where it belongs, of the right time and place. May it be a sound on the wind, enduring and clear, always. I thank you for this.*

# Love and Understanding

I heard a voice tonight on an answering machine, hard-edged, growing older quickly. I could feel the frustration, and could hear echoes of admonitions, "Jesus Christ, can't you see?" bouncing into my present. It's hard to talk about him, because the tenderness is so deep, and the mask over it so strong, the control so permanent. But it's all changing for him now. His kids are growing up, and his wife is saying no to what hasn't worked for her for years. He understands now, when she wears her guns and stands firm. She said she's been walking through his muck for years, holding only one foot on the path. This man of hers speaks with a firm lip and there is often fire in his eye.

He hasn't understood the depth of their needs to make their own decisions.

The best love I have had in a long time was simple. She said, "I am here," and stood looking at me with her weight on one foot, almost nonchalant, but quite serious. I tilted my head and looked at her, wondering if she knew what she was saying. It appeared she did, and so I stayed with her. It's been some time now, and she is still here. I think she understood what she saw.

I don't know why I ever bother to try to explain anything. I just get lost in all the connections and memories. What's the best truth is a description of the life I see around me. Everything buries itself in interpretations, changing connotations and contexts, and a million people stand on the street corners vending yesterday's knowledge. The fact is, knowledge itself is mercurial in my world. What stays is the desire to know, to stand under the rain of experience and let my love's eyes bathe me in quiet. It's because she wants this too that I allow it, and it's because she wants this that I am grateful.

Recently a woman stared at me across a coffee shop table with big dark eyes, staring without speaking, until I asked her, "What do you see?" She said she didn't know, so I asked her what she was looking for and she said, "I want to see who you are in my life." I thought that was pretty big stuff to catch with a long stare, so I said she could ask me. I thought I could answer her easy enough, because I knew it wasn't for me to give her what I began to feel she needed. I have fallen into the mother one too many times, and readily opt for something more balanced. There was a closing between us then, a rescinding of power into a face of kindness. Oh, my friend, how could you tender the world's pain in my heart? She didn't understand, because she seemed to think she did. It gets stuck so easily.

Soon I'll be landing on another continent, going back to the woman who said she was here, who still is, and my heart is fairly aching to sit with her in silence, and to listen to her tales, to smell the colors of her hair, to see the trails of her understanding ways passing before my eyes, always mobile, always new. We can't see the future, but it balloons before us like a fact of some kind we can't see the faces of. I know she sees, because she admits she hardly ever knows, and she always seems to be seeking, even when she orders me to come sit beside her to listen to the newest truth she has found. Always, there's a question in her eye, an opening for what is new, and this is what I know to be her love, like a child's vision in an adult mind and body, a child's soul looking out for splendor and magic, and for the truth these facets so easily engender. Control? No. Vision? Yes. She is the dreamer of this world to me, as I am her crazy dreaming man. We are kin. We understand each other. We are of the same wood.

This is the love we know, the kind that unfolds between us to be seen, the kind that always makes us new, even in all the years that may build between us. Respect is the base here, as we must constantly know it's being given to us on a daily basis, that neither of us creates anything alone, and that when we stand alone we stand inside the deepest lie ever told, and that when we try to form the other's life in our image we are fools to the core of our being, creating all that much more work to undo.

I must always listen, because understanding is always present; it just takes some time to get there, and a whole lot of patience when the opacity comes flying in robes of a thousand colors. It's like rain in the tropics sometimes, unexpected and intense, and who knows whether to take off the shirt and dance in it, or to run for cover. Listening gives the answer. I know I'm talking a good line, but these words are my own reminder and prayer. I'm asking that they stay with me when the shit comes raining down and the heart is lying shattered beneath stones of misunderstanding. Let me always wait to know. Let me always wait to see. In this we are all born clean.

## Traveler's Prayer

*You are with me always. I know this. This has been my life. You have never abandoned me, but always walked by my side. When I did not see you, you were by my side. Now I ask you to carry me far from my home, and let me find your ways there. Let my home grow beyond the sea, into the old lands, with the fathers from the other side of the world. Come with me in this journey. Lead me into this adventure. Let me live in your spirit still, though far from my lands. Let the spirit stretch. Please walk with me. I know your great love. Let my feet remain in your heart, my mind in your lungs. Let me breathe the spirit of your wisdom. Carry me in your arms to this next way. May the eyes of the hawk go with me, the mind of the coyote, the heart of the wind. May you be tender in my ways, Great One, and may I do your work wherever I go. May we never be broken. May we walk the medicine trail together through all time. In this I offer my life. In this I thank you for the gifts.*

# Berlin Wall

There is a low wall of ancient bricks, smiling faces, some grinning, some gesturing, hands reaching, pain across the countenance like a miming on a mountaintop, but the wall is in the middle of a city, and there are people dancing around it to a hard driving rhythm that keeps on and keeps on, spaces between sounds hitting sharp notes, staccato notes around the wall. A young girl sits on the wall, her legs dangling down, the backs of her calves touching the cold yellow-brown bricks. She looks at the ground, her countenance sad, then she looks skyward and her eyes pick up the light, but still there is a sadness there, a waiting for something, like a promise she was born with, a binding rope inside she is churning away from, and in this she sees a life of drama, of dance and music and living outside the boundaries of everything her parents knew as real that did not work for them. She does not show her anger, as it's been forbidden, but when the tears fall from her eyes, turning the bricks of the wall darker, she is not surprised. Nor is she upset, but instead a resolve begins to grow in her, as though watered by these tears, a resolve to be free, and to free the world at the same time, so she may be surrounded by freedom itself, understood, loved, held inside a world she can understand.

This wall is a monument to all the wars fought by civilizations strung out on themselves and their righteousness. Where is the patience in all this wounding? Where is the good? Who is not angry, and who can strike out at the one next to him without recoiling instantly? Who can we call to in the face of all this? Is love an answer to all this? Is the patience of the girl waiting on the wall, feet dangling, enough? Is ecstasy turning a corner in the world, peeking around the edge of reality into the living room of a peaceful home? It builds and builds, and we want to control it all forever, make it happen, rather than to wait and see what God has to offer us finally when all the shouting is done.

# Prayer in Germany

*Please let me see in time, this way to enter: let the joy be heard across the heart. It is huge. It is open sky, the heart that knows no bounds, circles spinning through time. Please may I always know the message of all gods. Let me see the stories. Even in this quiet they are speaking, marching across my mind from far in the past. I see the children wondering. I feel the radiation in the rain. Let me pull from all sources what needs to be said. Let me find more than the truth to give. Let me transform the sorrow we know. In this it may begin. May we all see what hurts and see the ways to gentleness. May we never cross the children's fire. Let this flame burn clean and free inside me always. In this I thank you for the life.*

# Workshops and the Butter Lady

There are almost too many things to talk about, to see, to reveal. There are the cruelties people turn away from, the concentration camps no one wants to visit, the prisons full of fancy wine and crystal glasses, and the tortures that bend people down deep inside, the external picture in a semblance of control. Here my anger tugs at me like a mean dog growling, and I don't know where to begin, how to tell of this in a way that does not build on itself to create an even worse monstrosity than what exists. What can be said? Is it fair to hold up a mirror to ugliness, or is it better to comb its hair and coo flattering words to it, soothing words to invite a change for the better? I don't really know. I know I care for these people, and that they live inside of me as surely as the crickets sing in the meadow tonight, asking for release.

I see a young expatriate woman in her room in a city in northern Italy, full of loneliness and change. Until recently she has been living in a long river valley full of careful fields and picturesque villages, under the steady gaze of ancient white glaciers. When I first met her there was a strong love begun between us immediately. As I sat at her sister-in-law's table and drank tea and wine, she gazed into my eyes without looking away. Her face was still, concentrated on gazing, then she burst into an uncontrollable smile of recognition. I was surprised that no one else related to her obvious joy, as though she were a mental patient, almost slightly invisible. I discovered later that she had just been released from a local hospital, having suffered physical results of what she described as chronic depression. Altogether, the situation and feeling was very strange. Her husband asked her, in very polite tones, to fetch something from the kitchen, and she sobered herself and went to the task. When it was accomplished she sat again, and stared into my eyes. I felt like a hero in an old swashbuckling movie, like a good pirate in disguise in the powerful lord's den. Her husband's smile was cold and distant from her, yet warm and inviting to me. I made arrangements to visit them again later in the month, and to stay for a few days. When I said goodbye she hugged me very close, and I knew that there would be another powerful exchange between us, something elemental.

When I returned weeks later, I was told upon entering that she was not feeling well, and would be down after awhile. I was invited to have tea, but

I declined and went upstairs instead. When I entered her bedroom, knocking lightly, she leaned up from her position on the bed, where she had been curled up in a long dark miasma, her skin yellow. Her eyes opened wide, and I smiled to her. She ran to me, threw her arms around me and repeated over and over, "You're here, you're really here. You really came back." She wept freely, and held me with all her strength. I carried her to the bed and held her quietly, stroking her softly, then after some time of calming, began to rub her feet and legs. Eventually I rubbed her entire body softly, and she cried and laughed for a long time.

Until this time we had hardly spoken with each other, so the next day we went into the mountains and I heard her story. It was about a marriage, a love affair her husband had begun before the marriage, and the blossoming of this affair now, years later. It included much suffering in between. She said nothing bad about her husband, yet it was apparent to me that she was deeply oppressed, her feelings being denied in fundamental ways. She had allowed the affair, ostensibly out of love for her husband, as a sort of gift to him, but was unaware of the problems this would cause for her. She was young, and he was her teacher, so she set her own needs aside. The problems involved screaming matches and vows of hatred in the street, twisted visions of her desires and place in the family. She was living something contradictory to her heart, the greatest omission, the greatest fall from grace.

I listened to her story for hours, asking many questions. Although I have seen many such situations, and have lived in the center of different forms of this myself, there was a quality of contradiction here that was difficult to fathom. There was an unwitting cruelty at base that fascinated me, and I could not let her fall prey to it any longer. She had seen me in a way that I could not deny, and I had simply recognized her. I had done little else but that, and that was enough to explode through her life. What a prison she must have endured.

Later I saw the forms of it. Her sister-in-law made comments in front of her. "Oh you don't know her. When you get to know her better you'll find she's not so smart." Her husband's kind face was so closed off from loving her that it hurt me to see it, too much protection from the truth of his responsibility in her life obscuring anything but techniques for transforming pain. Perhaps he was as confused as her, but he was not in the hospital, in any case.

Why would she want to transform the pain, rather than the situation that caused it? She sought to live for seven years under a law her husband laid down, one of evolution of the consciousness past suffering, in a situation of consummate suffering, and she believed his ways, not seeing how he was protecting himself from personal responsibility. In so doing, she became a willing slave, dominated by a picture of how she should be, of how modern, how illuminated and allowing. The more I lived with them the more horrified I became. I witnessed countless moments of abuse, times when she swallowed her treatment without screaming out.

The mode in the home was one of higher mind. There were crystals and a million patterns of understanding. The husband, another expatriate, was a very bright young counselor beginning to evolve psychic gifts, who spent much time looking into the depths of reality in workshops and private meditation of his own style. His counseling manners were very positive and comforting to begin with, yet I found that once he established a confidence, he began to work on "problems." As I sat in session with him I found his approach to be fascinating, his mind quite complex and circuitous in an entertaining way, until he came suddenly to the notions of problems, without any agreement that this was going to be a focus between us. At that point I began to look at his motives with an objective eye. I began to see the whole of his life, and to find once again how important it is that someone in his position have a strong base of support around him. The fact that his wife was in great pain that he did little to alleviate gave him reason enough to hide from me, and gave me reason enough to be suspicious of his abilities to counsel. The sudden and unforeseen move to 'problems' shifted the base of trust, and his own pattern of seeing the world began to emerge. Control became the issue, and I saw the roots of his dominance. His "inner voice" became important, and he began to explain concepts in rudimentary manners without seeing that I already understood them. Style began to dominate the substance of what was between us, and I became a mirror of his ego. All positions were lost at that point for me, everything gone into a slippery realm where I knew I had to travel to see what was there. What had begun as enjoyment became a battle between power and perception. It is fascinating how quickly the most crucial issues emerge, how easily we dive beneath the surface of things to see the wild forces of life wielding battle axes and swirling vortexes like out of comic books, just to maintain ignorance and ways that don't work for everyone involved. In such situations I feel there is little for me to do but to ask questions and stay in the center of everything as best I can.

To make the change between the young woman and myself, we climbed a waterfall in the rain. We ran out of talk, into the center of her depression, where she could not move, but only stand shivering in the wet, not being able to take another step. We stood together at the base of the fall, its sound merciless, the cloud of mist enveloping us, filling us with its chill and strength. She began to be vitalized. We climbed to the top of the fall, winding our ways through the wet forest, bright red mushrooms along the path, with fern glens, animal spoor, and steady rain. At the top we found a rock bed alongside the stream at the point where it leaped over the edge. We laid on our backs in transparent raincoats, opening our faces to the sky. Three great waterfalls poured down into the valley where we lay, seeming to come from the sky itself. I took a small stone from the stream and held it to the sky. Clouds rose up from the ground, and there was a great joining of vapor and water and sound all around us. I held the stone high for a long while, praying, and I felt all the ancestors join us there, the sisters from the south, the old ones from the west; every good force I'd ever known in my life joined us there as she cried into the rain. I cried to watch her, our tears running down our faces in rainwater. I could feel it all pouring out of her, the years of pain, the fear of where she must go inside her strength to move onward. I gave her the river stone, and she washed it with stream water, kneeled and prayed for a long while. I moved into the trees to give her privacy. She came to me when she was finished, smiled, kissed my cheek, held me, and began laughing. The rain smelled like salt in her hair, and we ran down the mountain laughing. Each time we looked at each other there was great laughter, and we ran through the stream leaping high into the air and splashing rain everywhere.

That afternoon we drove up out of the valley to visit a farmhouse to buy butter for the evening meal. The butter lady was a heavy woman who stood strongly on the Italian soil without a trace of insecurity about anything, greeting us with a smile as broad as her face, a smile of deep intelligence and humor. She embraced the young woman with deep respect, and an eye that saw everything about her, everything that happened that day, penetrating deeply, completely unafraid. She looked as though she owned the earth, and the earth owned her at the same time. She shook my hand strongly, and I felt I had met a friend, a person I could trust solidly. There was an instant camaraderie, and when I looked at my companion I saw an incredible strength and clarity in her, as though she was at home in herself in a way I hadn't seen before. She fairly shone, and her laughter contained a deep wisdom, as though her suffering had suddenly become something else, powerfully defined into compassion. I wanted to talk with the butter lady, but she spoke only Italian, of which I knew virtually nothing, so we agreed to talk only with our eyes. She told the young woman it would have to do for now, and I heartily agreed. It was more than enough against the backdrop of all the sorrow we had seen those days.

We visited for an hour, with me listening to the rhythms of their talk dance across the valley, watching chickens scratch in the yard. Clouds rolled in over the snow-topped peaks and I began to feel at home.

When we left I wanted to visit more farmers, so we did, and everywhere we went I noticed the young woman's carriage, her erect but easy posture, the dignity with which she was met, and the grace in which she carried herself. A beauty emerged through the afternoon that made me deeply happy, and I felt all would be well with her. At one point we perched on an outcropping of rock looking towards the southern fields and spoke about workshops and meditation and consciousness. We were irreverent about such things, though respectful in our own ways, and we decided that the butter lady was by far the most enlightened person we had seen in years. There were no secrets about her, no hidden agendas, no pocketbooks to fill or spiritual egos to assuage. As I thought back on the whole thing, I was sure this was true, and the ease she imparted to how we breathed and took in life was contagious beyond description. Her parting hug to my friend was long and strong amidst the clucking chickens and bright sunlight, and we agreed we would all see each other again to talk about life in much the same way as we had that day. We were all free, and obliged to keep it that way between us as long as possible. We understood the obligations of love.

Later there was a long conversation with her husband about sensitivity. We wrestled through convolutions of understanding that masked feelings held for centuries, a long unmet male tradition, until there began to be a breakthrough and he said he finally began to feel the world around him. He said he felt more responsive to people around him than ever before. His wife watched in amazement, a smile on her face, a quiet smile full of trepidation, yet of joy, relief and expectation. Then he said the hours of our talk made him feel closer than ever to his lover, and as he said this, his wife caved in, as though kicked in the stomach. Her skin paled and her lips quivered, and I felt she might become sick, but I watched, supporting her with my gaze. She held my eyes desperately, hardly believing what she was hearing. He looked at me, only glancing slightly toward his wife. Then he turned to face her, and repeated his words, leaving me incredulous, having seldom seen such emotional cruelty. I have seen people call one another the most vile names, victimize one another physically and emotionally, mentally in every way possible, yet there was something so absent in his manner with her that I was appalled. How could he not see what he was doing to her? But I said nothing. I waited, and when she looked to me I said, "Are you seeing what you need to see?" She nodded, then excused herself and left the table. After a short while, with no acknowledgment of what he had done, he went to tend to her. It didn't last long and he returned to tell me she wanted to talk with me. He told me to be sure and get a good night's sleep, not to talk too long, to take care of myself. His sister seconded his comment and told me the young wife could go on all night long, and to be sure to take care of myself. This was obviously the mode in these relationships.

Her first words when I entered the room were, "I don't think I can spend another day in this crazy house." I nodded and raised my eyebrows. I held her hand and we drifted into sleep.

Power was the dynamic here, honesty the deception. It was fine for him to be honest with his feelings about his lover, but it was not acceptable that she be devastated. She must leave her suffering behind. His desires were considered to be a condition of truth she must be strong enough to endure. Strength of character must be developed at all costs, at the cost of personal dignity, at the cost of self-respect. She loved me immediately, without fear, with passion, and with an ability to be close and sure, while he held me at a distance of understanding, in the realms of mindful fascination, a brotherhood of knowing. There was genuine affection between us, and between them as well, but the desire for personal power, and the belief in personal power as an end, buried all sense of active compassion. Cruelty ran rampant, out of control, blindness everywhere smashing tenderness into oblivion.

I can't turn away from these pictures, though I desperately pray for resolution, for her strength and his illumination, for he is in a position of much power in the world, and has many people who believe in his abilities, who count on him for help. Yet I know where the illusions will take him, and where her heart will take her. It is only the matter of in-betweens that concern me, and of the influences that will occur. The echoes of his running are loud, and come from all those around him, and the intrinsic quietness of her soul is profound. It is a statement of the world that these people stand as they do, the meek and the powerful, and where the meek endure, and the powerful burst at the seams, running through their darkness alone. Yet there is a benevolence in all of this for everyone, that quietly churns in the center of it. It is an unveiling, an old dance bringing an eventual peace. I know this, and I see shadows of it emerging. I hear the counselor begin to teach the knowledge she has given him, and I wonder if he can acknowledge its source. I wonder what he knows. Can he get out of the way enough to let his gentleness speak? Can he begin to care for his wife, though everything is changing?

Now she is living in a small town with a river running through it, listening to the music of revolution on her cassette player. One of the sisters from the south sent her a primer on women's liberation she said made her laugh gratefully, with its obvious applications to her life. She bought a plant some weeks ago for her first apartment, and is looking at a Toulouse-Lautrec painting in bright colors. She is alone, lonely, and full of sorrow, yet when we spoke last she told me that if I ever needed anything to call her. She said she was sending strength to me through the air. I feel it now, as I seek to find meaning in all this darkness. She is with me as I speak these words. I see her walking along the river by herself in the evening, reflecting on all these changes. She told me on the phone that she has been meeting many butter ladies where she works, and that it's a good thing there are so many around.

## Prayer to Find the Silence

*There is a space between that waits, like a cat for the evening meal, motionless in the field, beginning finally to look like a fixture of the landscape, a dry branch in the shape of a waiting cat. And when it's time, the lightning is there, without tension or reflection, but sudden and sure, something given from nature that endures and provides. Let silence give to us in this way, whatever it contains. Let it stand ready beside us like an excited angel, bursting with information. Let it alleviate sadness by providing an open field of possibilities, of dreams that don't have to go away. Let it provide an evening of pleasure across the chest, sinking into the next day. And when the noise is too much, let this silence make a quiet brain, handing down one thing at a time, wrapped in gold lights or promises of fulfillment. Let it at least give a moment of adventure in all the knowing, a suddenness that's relief against predictability. It gets to be too much any other way. Please let this be, amongst all the other ways you have to reach us.*

# Silent Anger

Sometimes I'm so angry it turns the sun away, makes him hide somewhere like a frightened animal. Sometimes I feel such a despair that I could wither in a frightening manner, or explode across the face of the earth. Then there is little to do but wait, though I might see a woman to nurture me, to hold me and assuage this tyranny of feeling.

I might see a life of control ahead of me, of discipline and regularity, predictability, clocking into one day after another. I see myself smoking a pipe then, breathing in through my nostrils before I say something profound, and I know what bullshit this is. I look at all the men I know, and I think about what I respect. It isn't knowledge, or talent, or awareness, but more it's courage, tenderness, and an ability to care, to respond. I want to reach out and grab so many of my brothers by the scruffs of their necks and stand in their faces. Fuck your talent, I want to scream, and fuck your genius and your awareness and your fat ass sense of your self. Get off it and look around you. You don't know anything if you can't take care of the people around you.

But I don't say these things, because I think it's not my place. I let the pieces fall where they may, and I only expose what I see might help. For me it's a quiet revolution that goes the deepest, but sometimes I can't stand it, and I want to rip the facade off style and grace and decency and elegance and lay it bare before a man's soul.

It's easy to see sometimes, almost too easy. I stand back and fight the depression inside myself, as I'm his brother, and I turn to make a piece of the world I can live with, feeling like the lone ranger. Keys begin to emerge, and I realize I have to be with those who see, and if there are none, then I have to be here in the middle of the night piecing all this together to say what is at base. It isn't what I want that matters. It's what's at base but gets crushed that's so sorrowful. It's what we all seem to want but what we let be stifled, smothered, and made blind that's so deeply lost. It's a cry that comes from our own throats a surprise, a sound that leaps into being without preconception in the night, something we only look at for a brief second before we turn away. It's lost then, but never disappears. It's what we know is true, and that which we believe we cannot live.

# Life Prayer

*Oh dear Lord I see myself by firelight, smiling out of the darkness, and I think back on the times of not knowing, of my ignorance and fear, my creeping desires to pad back into the life I could always only see from a distance, the marriage and the job, the steadiness of the blind eye, the security of not knowing even more than I do now. You grin at my words tonight. I can see your smile and hear your chuckle, but I shake my head in bewilderment. I want back into being sure of what it all means, back out of the magic, the quick dives into the slippery realms where you live and build the beginnings of life. As I have found you here waiting for me, and as I seek to do your work, I begin to understand how this could never be told from the outside, how there could be knowing only from here, yet this is all as familiar as coming home from a long journey. It is a mystery unveiled to be more mysterious than ever. I live beyond what my imagination could have contrived, and the simplicity is full of humor, a young man's face laughing, incredulous in the beginnings of freedom. "It's simple," he said. "Isn't it? It's simple." Over and over he repeated this, and it doesn't leave me, but piles up with all the history. Perhaps I never would have begun, if I had known a choice. And perhaps this is a useless conjecture. I hear you laughing.*

*But what will you do with me now that you have me on this beautiful spinning wheel of yours? I am completely out of answers, out of questions, and my mind is quickly turning vagabond on the landscape of my people's imagination. I need you as never before. Please fill me tenderly. I am an open wound spread across your sky, willing but afraid. Fill me gently, and when you are done with me, please take me home to sleep. From somewhere in my existence I feel my bones dissolve into your vast sweetness, and I am already tired. I hope it is not too soon.*

# Motive

I listen to distant drumming on a cold dark night and speak to the ancestors. Patches of snow dot rolling hills and the air goes straight into the center of my bones. I listen, in need again.

I don't know how to live anymore without this call. I have to be in the middle of time in order to be at full strength, in order to have the calm view. I have to call back in time for assistance, in order to move into the future with balance. This call is a reaching out into the air around me, opening my hands and mind and senses into the quiet dimension just outside of conversations at the dinner table, the dimension where a gentle knowing waits leaning on its side, head resting against an open palm, smiling.

Sometimes it's a somber image, one from another race of people, and sometimes it's a fierce warrior's face that looks at me from the darkness. They are all a continual presence waiting, watching, speaking, listening, doing all the things that I do, but just a notch over into the unexpected, into a deep step of friendliness, like the waiting arms of a guardian angel.

I have needed them lately, because the work has become a bit different. Some people have been describing my appearance while I work, and what I look like afterward. They say I'm glowing, that I look ageless and very peaceful. This is understandable, because it's like a sauna for me, not in the sense of direct heat, but as a way of cleansing.

I've been having to clarify my motives again and again, and this takes me into a very deep place in myself, as I see things operating in people that I do not like, ways of deceit that spread out to hurt those around them, ways that are hurting the people themselves most obviously. Within this, I have to retain my own value system while working, yet I must stay true at the same time to the value of healing as the first priority, without stopping anywhere. It can't be a matter of judgment and condemnation, but more of a judgment that occurs in perceiving what there is to deal with. In this I see a thousand stances of morality, immorality, and amorality, each called the other at different times in order to facilitate the individual's needs. These notions are all rather slippery and adaptable to a particular moment. This has always seemed to be the case, what with religious wars righteously fought against infidels, and now people are doing the same thing in the name of spreading enlightenment to the world, not seeing the nature of the usury they create around them. The infidel lies within the heart of the crusader.

What I often see specifically in a person is the lie, or the crying child, a mother or father scolding cruelly in the background, an old chair or a bed present off to the side, and perhaps a picture from a photo album of a child with a frightened and grim face. I might be holding a person's liver when I see this, so I speak quietly to the child I see, telling him it's going to be all right, that he can come along without so much fear, that he'll be taken care of, integrated into the whole person. Then he might turn into a petulant little bastard, so I'll speak harshly to him, telling him to get his shit together and get onto his own whole truth and stop hanging around punishing everyone else for his history.

Sometimes I find a jaw muscle tied up with telling an old lie, and I see this clearly, what the lie is, that it is, how long its been going on, and how it keeps the person alive in a style to which he's become accustomed. When I work it loose, I have to pray for a gentle seeing, because lies are powerful things in the body, and the next step, where it finally releases from the tissue into the blood, has to be dealt with on every level, from electro-magnetic connections in the nerves and muscles, to the fluid in the tissues, to the extra load on the heart and organs that dealing with the traveling garbage entails.

I keep finding that in this proliferation of activities I can only ask for help, because it takes a strong will and a deep acceptance on the part of the person I'm working on to deal with old unseen habits, especially if they are destructive. People are loath to see these things. It seems we get used to dying a certain way, calling it living, and the nature of the dance we do is absolute reality to us. The longer its been going on, the stronger it is, seeking always to perpetuate itself. We can even call it talent, and one strong arm of it might just be that, while the whole creature seen all together is just a raging beast creating an empire quickly going nowhere with a great flourish.

These things make it very difficult to talk with anyone about this kind of work. It's too much, and anything I might say could easily be construed the wrong way. I even hesitate to say these words, but feel a need to record the phenomenon for later understanding, and for clarification right now. It's a reminder to myself that I have to be intact.

I see shit I don't like to see, and I can't change this, but must deal with it. I have to handle my own anger in order to turn bullshit into chicken bones, and ancient lies into corn cobs, so they might be removed, and when dark forces come lurking out of kidneys I sometimes feel the need to throw spears before I can pull strength from a powerful enduring heart to fill the void. I feel myself to be a reluctant warrior in this place, yet I see what must be done for the well-being of the person in my hands, and there is a deep trust to be honored between us. I cannot limit my vision of the person to any one strange part, but must see the potential, the depth of what is there, the underpinnings, and feel the presence of benevolence as well as the destruction. Together they make the whole person, and that's what I'm dealing with.

This is where the help comes in. Everyone's history is bigger than my knowledge of it, my interpretation of it, or my ability to perceive where it must go, though I might sense the fact that something must occur. At best, I can only wish the best for the person, and for all those around him. So in this light, I continually ask that a greater will than my own be done. Again in this light, it follows that it must be a greater will than the person's as well, in order that he might gain entry into the next steps of himself. If he does not allow this, he will not move, but will only find his expectations, fears, and limitations staring him in the face. He will not get permanently well, but will bang against the walls of himself interminably, going back and forth with his healing process. It isn't a hierarchy or a linear progression, but a matter of simultaneous connections between the body, the mind, the heart, the history, and most importantly, the desire, and this can only be greater than what the person knows. The person himself must deeply acknowledge both sides of himself and allow himself to be truly seen by others. If he maintains that others only see his good side, it won't work. As he seeks to fool others, he fools himself, and this goes both directions in a vicious circle.

So I ask for lots of help, both from my own god, and from all of his as well, from those I can name, and from all the nameless forces of goodness that surround us constantly waiting for recognition.

It is in this way that I take time to listen to the gods of this old land tonight to court their favor, to ask for their knowledge and strength, while a wind howls through cold pines. There are many traditions alive here that resist inevitable changes, and the ghosts of wars churn everywhere, til there is a steady humming of them in the brain. Because of this, there is much running away, and much anger, with huge amounts of inertia. Things here are very deeply not what they seem, and power reigns over the people as they sleep. Freedom remains in the realm of prayers, and there are empty churches everywhere.

## Prayer to the Teutonic Gods

*Do I know you, old ones? Do I remember you, and are you still in my blood too? Or is it too late? What is this crying that I hear, and where is the center of the stillness that I feel? Can you teach the ghosts to sing, or is it that they must remind us of what we do not want to remember? I don't know anymore, but I feel you, and see you staring from the eyes of children. I hear you deep in the woods, where even the animals seem to read books to know themselves, this land has been so long full of people. I can see your shadows, and sometimes your fierce eyes, sometimes embarrassed eyes, sometimes an eternal patience glowing from behind a tree, or a gentle arm reaching around from behind a winter branch. Is it you who make this stark landscape, like a moon valley built for pondering? Are you a thousand separate arms of your Father, quiet in your business of building bridges across time, season after season? I listen for you, and ask your help now. I have touched this ground with questions, these people with love, and I am left not knowing, more than usual. Please come into my dreams with care, and take me to my waiting Mother. Come from antiquity to take me home, and bring the deepest healing from everywhere in between. Please come do this tonight, under the bright song of the cold church bell, and when you have done this, let my love hold me close in her arms. I admit my spirit is tired, and I need your help here now.*

# Dilemmas

I was in a car with a brother who teaches awareness for a living, one man among many these days.
He tells his students that as their consciousness
moves downward into their bodies, they become
more deeply rooted with the earth, and with the
universality of human connection, feeling at one
with their brothers and sisters across time and cultural barriers. A deep peace emerges as one feels
this connection with our common roots, he maintains. He has a strong conviction that spreading this
consciousness will bring world peace, superceding
political action, and that he, along with many others, is at the cutting edge of a great leap forward in
the development of mankind. His life is devoted to
this task, and he works long hours promoting his
project, traveling the globe to realize his dream.

All this came to my mind like a spring bubbling
up out of the ground as we sat in a car together,
waiting to get into traffic. An older man was in a car
in front of us, a bright red rental car that under-
scored the man's fragility behind the wheel. He was

clearly out of his element. My brother kept inching
forward, with an intense look about him, coming
alongside the man, finally edging him out of position, intimidating him without looking into his face.
I could only imagine the feeling in the man's heart.
He looked to be from a small town in the Midwest,
far from home, far from his own sense of security.
My brother edged out others coming from the front
as well. In the middle of these actions, which took
some time, I asked him where he was going, and he
said "I'm going to be the first one on the road." I
wondered what road he meant, and felt I didn't
want to be on it with him. The trade-off was too
deep. People hollered at him as he pulled into traffic.

We live such contradictions. I felt at a loss as to
how to handle the situation because the dominance
and misplaced aggression was so obvious, and the
contradiction so deep. My brother felt like a stranger
to me then. He was punishing someone for something obscure.

Later, outside one of his classes, I was asked by
a participant to help get her car started. She had
called a tow truck, but wanted to save some money,
so I helped her, messing with greasy jumper cables
in the dark. I did so simply because I could, because
she had asked, and because I've appreciated the
help others have given me. It was just the right
thing to do. Throughout the time I was with her the
woman moved quickly, though she was slightly on

the heavy side, and her eyes darted off to the side easily. I wondered where her mind was.

When we got her car going, she was ready to take off without calling the tow truck operator to let him know she didn't need him, something which surprised me. It seemed a matter of course to her. Why couldn't she see that the driver might be a man like me, one who had just helped her? It certainly wasn't a stretch to see this. I pictured the driver arriving, being unable to find her, calling back in to the office to see if he'd screwed up the directions, going through the anxiety of missing her, losing his time and gas, and then his faith when it finally became apparent that she had simply left. Would he treat the next person like shit to compensate? Would the old man in the red car bark at his wife to regain his sense of power, or would he wither silently in his own way and add this small incident to his declining belief in the young? I wondered to myself what the woman had learned in a six hour class about getting in touch with herself. There was no softness present and the chain of events she was willing to put into place was obviously thoughtless, without consideration of outcome. I wondered where the universality of man had disappeared to for both of these people.

Perhaps my brother is not responsible for his student's actions, but every minute of every day we are each given options of what we can contribute, and we make choices, no matter what we might say. We all make errors in judgment, but when we have time to think, or to answer the question of where we are going, why step on the stranger? Does he represent the face of the enemy? Is he less than anyone else, unworthy of respect because he is not known? Is he invisible, or is he the competitor? Because my brother works hard in his own field does this give him the right to ignore another's? Has the golden rule become "Do unto others before they do unto you?"

The most compassionate view I can find regarding these small kinds of incidents is to see the ways in which diseases and preoccupations with the self blind one person from another. Sometimes development of the self creates even more isolation than there was to begin with, and lack of a sense of community, and both these incidents seemed evidence of this. It's difficult to see the outside world while looking in a mirror. And, there can be many biochemical factors seen when looking at values and lapses of consciousness that are very real as well. There are a thousand reasons.

The whole world is a living breathing creature, and scenes like this continually spur me on to working harder to move beyond my own obscurities. I can't ignore them. These moments propel me into a deep sadness, where my faith reaches far beyond my brother for what I need to live by, into some eternal law of retribution and balance, where everything comes back around the way it began, only bigger and with another face. What allows this is again something gargantuan, like an unmoving eye that never blinks, but only watches and watches, without judgment, without reaction, impassive, enduring and ominous.

## Prayer for Dealing with Bullshit

*Dear Lord let me steer clear of bullshit, and when it rains down let me not be afraid, but wary, seeing, and compassionate. I want to see who and where the bulls are, inside and outside, and I cannot stay where it's always going in one direction, where I must be patient all the time, where the listening is always work. It's true I want joy, and trust, and with these things I will pass through places of usury. Let me be free in my own counsel, and release me from any obligations to illuminate truth, and let the truth be known still. I must trust in you, finally, and that your desire will come to life, eventually. It's always a matter of time, and in this my own freedom lies. Let my anger protect me and those I love, and do nothing more. Let me be discreet. Let the bullshit fall where it becomes obvious, and let me step around it easily. There is only so much time, and I'm getting too old for this.*

# A Note on Healing

It doesn't matter what the points connected with are, as long as the connection is clean and once again, the motive clear. The whole connection will get the juice where it needs to go, and the best connection is at the easiest point of entry, one freely given and found in comfort of the spirit. I must avoid a system because it's too slow and it becomes "mine" too easily. This is still another reminder, the same one I keep hearing over and over.

I have to stay clear with myself that I go beyond the role of healer into that of the friend. This is where I want to be. I'm no professional, and belong to no circle. Circles and inner circles, and core groups as concepts, run contrary to my world view. Looking back on this in my life, I find that every time I've entered a circle it's proven to be more isolating than my life likes to be. There's a danger in this concept, as there can be in concepts in general, and this is ironic, as I am in love with ideas, but the attitude of owning them is a sore temptation I wish to avoid. I always come down to knowing that vision itself produces the most efficient way of being in the world, the act and the art, the vision of listening and seeing. I see that this mode empowers all those around me as well, and spreads my world outward to include a great many people, though certainly not everyone. There are those who don't like to be seen, and my vision is not always clear itself.

But how is the effectiveness of a teacher or healer measured? This is a huge thing to answer, and I'm as lost as anyone else in this maze of living, though I have directions and values I believe in. There is a tension between the flesh and the spirit, between the real and the imagined, that drives many people into stasis, out of fear, but it's an essential tension, a method by which we live, and wants to be embraced passionately. I want those I come in contact with to become well, strong and productive in their own eyes, not in mine, though it's not at all important if they know exactly what's going on. If a person's sick, I want him well, and I feel my clarity in this desire to be the primary key to helping. I won't accept money for what I do because it's no profession, and I want no expectations on whatever connection might be found between me and someone else. I don't want anything involving buying and selling in this ground.

Something is lost in this exchange and I know I don't have anything to offer that's guaranteed.

Often I see physical problems that are indirect results of an imbalance in the value system. This is a touchy area, because values run deep and people seldom want to change them. They've gotten a person so far, so why change them? It's scary business, with no known outcome. But this may be where the action is, where the deepest healings are allowed to happen, because a person is willing to re-examine everything, every part of life, if he'll look at his values. In this basic meeting the chances for progressing are best, because a principle that may be obscure by virtue of its size and power could appear minuscule and easily revealed to be powerless in another context, from another value. In a way this is the same idea that it doesn't matter what point on the body one begins with, as long as the entry is comfortable for both people involved. It's a shift in vision that wants to be simple, almost experimental. The assumption is simple. A man recently asked me, as I was working on his knees and shins during an asthma attack, what the connection was between the legs and lungs. I thought for a moment, then answered "It's the same body." Cute? No. It's just true. I couldn't take the time to go into stuff about organs and nerves and blood systems and grounding. What did either of us need to know but that his body was coming together to breathe again?

I seem to know less and less, and more and more at the same time. In this some things are painfully obvious. For example, someone may develop a great system for healing, creative and dynamic, alive and full, and he may carry it for years, until it begins to grow beyond itself, while the creator, the discoverer, still hangs onto how it began. He can't see how it needs to change, how it needs to feed more people, to create broader support for others in order to continue growing without eating him alive. He might find himself wondering at what is going wrong as he is more and more dissatisfied with the performance of those around him, asking of others the same intensity he asks of himself, but without affording them the same vision in all the terms he knows, without affording them the same security. He may wonder what is going wrong with his body, as all this surfaces in that form. It may all come down to an imbalanced distribution of a growing power.

The inability to make the change at this point has destroyed many a genius, and many a high powered businessman. In the healing world, this dynamic is especially powerful because the notions of what healing is are often involved with a large sense of community, and sense of the oneness of all living creatures, and without this living in a visceral sense there can be big trouble. Without integrating the life with the teaching, destruction will ensue.

A man may pick a viewpoint, call it his own, and tell what he sees with the authority of what is real. It's clear to him, and the revelation may well have saved his life at one time. But then the process changes as it moves out into the public eye and the person becomes an expert, the voice of a theory, of an inspiration. It's born, then taught, sold in the marketplace of education, and another force begins to operate that takes the founder away from the roots of discovery and into the jaws of production. He must go forward and upward or sink, in his eyes. What was born in a realization of universal community then begins to become solitary by virtue of ownership, and begins to separate the person from the original impulse to join the world on the world's terms. It becomes rigid. The maestro then wants to change the world, to meet it only on his terms, an endeavor full of danger and peaceful-looking arrogance. The balance here is hard to find, and the voice speaking often overrides the voices listened to. Underneath the calm face, a cyclone rages.

This becomes a picture of isolation, finally, and ironically, because it is usually in intense isolation that the original sense of unity was found. There is nothing left but to join, or to realize what is already joined when one is over his own edge into the beyond.

With isolation the circle comes complete for this person. He finds himself alone again, his greatest fear, but on a much more powerful level, one that threatens the destruction of the entire world he has built up. But one may have secretly desired this state in his drive to become immersed in the crucible again, in the purity of intense loneliness, the fire of knowing at the edge of existence. Unfortunately, he may not recognize that this drive is at the core of his style. It may be one crucial pattern that hasn't changed in his life, something born in childhood and never left behind.

Someone once told me that "we do what we know," and it fit the situation I was in at the time perfectly. I'd been wondering what I was going to do next with my life. It's fit a thousand times since then, one of those Zen Biblical expressions that finishes off circular wonderings around the plight of our ideas and need to accomplish something, with a simple nod. It would appear that the only freedom in the midst of all this is to continue looking, trying to see the way clear, weaving in and around the patterns being lived so furiously.

The casualties in all this are those who climb onto another's train without seeing the cliff over which it must inevitably plunge. They think they're on a beautiful ride, full of power and grandeur, then when the change comes, there's not a tool for survival in sight, and the trade-off they've made is hollow, and they have to find their own way in the darkness, all alone in what could be a very sad beginning.

# Desperation Prayer

*I'm tired inside, depleted, love everywhere, but a deep wounding coming to the surface, a tethered goat buried deep inside of me. I'm turning circles in the hot sun. Please bring me the voice I can hear, the eyes to speak to. Oh Lord come into me quietly tonight; my spirit is asleep, groggy and too far from elation. You say to find the gentle fire. Yes. I listen, distant tears always attendant, yet I am impatient and want to know it all right now. Curl up with me tonight and breathe into my ear, Kali. All you women, grab me by the hair and drag me laughing across the moonless sky. I cannot find purpose, and the truth has no luster. There is only the faith that has accumulated these last years. It will take me to bed alone, perhaps to give me a dream of love. But I am even too tired to dream, and I barely beseech you with this indulgence. Wrap me in your gentleness tonight, four winds, and take me home quietly. I am afraid of your stillness. Let this not last my life.*

*Oh God fill me with fire please. I only have so much time, and there is so much I must do. I must tend to these people, and to that truth, and to this delicacy, this gentleness which needs to grow and live beyond obscurity. Give me time please Lord, to burst these chains, to fill to* spilling over. Let me live in your voice, and speak the words of your desire. In this I ask for the dream to come true. Oh please Lord take me home before my time is over. I am yours in desperation.

## Prayer to Move Through Darkness

*It's everywhere. Take me through no matter what, when the whirling begins, and put me in the forest awhile to listen to the biggest truth. Don't let me be caught in anyone's chaos unaware, voices screaming on the inside, but set me under the spell of trees' quiet talking. Let the cold night air shake me alive then, and let the shadows be full only with the murmurings of peaceful night creatures. Slow me down to listen and to feel again, to know my place in your heart.*

# Dreams

I had a nightmare last night without a doubt, one that challenged my faith, a crazy too-sane complex dream that my love turned away from me. It was an exagerrated mirroring of little things, built into a monster experience that left me depressed on waking. I wrote a description of it and my feelings which I mistakenly read at breakfast, and witnessed the fears manifest in her, then me, then her, like a ping-pong ball bouncing off stones. I regretted I'd shared it. It made me light six candles in a six hundred year old church to pray, cold bright light streaming through stained glass scenes of workers rising above struggle, conquering evil. It made me look again at what dreams are and how I relate to them.

When I was a kid fluorescent blue crabs used to go after my feet and I'd wake up no bigger than my pillow, every inch of me at the head of my bed. Then as I grew older a few existential nightmares came in and I saw the world destroyed by man-eating slugs, creatures that would dissolve everything but the soul. In those dreams I saw Heaven, all white, and myself as a baby just born. God told me I could watch my life this time around. Okay. I've been trying to do just that. This was a heavy dream with a good ending.

Interspersed with these dreams were some concentration camp nightmares, the same dream over and over, in which I was shot but not killed, and ended up escaping naked into the woods around Dachau. This was an old one, very graphic, that made me look deeply into Man's potential for controlled insanity, a narcissistic attitude gone to its mad conclusion. I have seen this in all cultures, and came to terms with it after finally spending a day in Dachau, peering into the ovens and listening to the visitors crying.

As I matured my nightmares became mostly limited to good-versus-evil scenarios, and sometimes dealt with space creatures who impassively slaughtered all humans. In these dreams my palms emanated a bright white light like a ray, that would blast the creatures' ships out of the sky. At intense moments I would tilt my head back and utter a warbling cry, like a war cry, that called up all the powers around me to do battle. Once one of the space ships flew up to me during a battle, eye level, and a keyboard slid out toward me that looked familiar, and I punched in a few numbers, and the battle stopped.

This was a pre-computer-age dream, and now I wish it was all that easy.

The power in the hands came up in several other repeating dreams, and was always coupled with the warbling cry. My sleeping companion said it was intense and other-worldly, like from another time, but that it caused no fear at all.

All these dreams were certainly not predominant in my dream life. Most dreams have been good, the sexual ones in a very loving way, many of complex interrelations between people, and many of flying, and being transformed into light, this kind of thing. It's been the gamut of dream life.

What I've come to feel is that different levels of dreaming happen, that some are pictures of today's reality put in another way, easier to deal with sometimes, sometimes more complex, so as to produce intrigue, perhaps, or at least another way to see what's going on. Some are magnifications of fear, and provide a deep experience of something that's been nagging at the psyche. If we look at these we can come to understand ourselves better, regardless of whether the dream is resolved or not. There are a million ways to interpret dreams, with symbols on top of symbols, and many complex languages have been developed to unravel the mysteries of dream consciousness. They are fascinating tools, all of the ones I've encountered.

Another way of dreaming is that it is just like living awake. It's an experience, not open to interpretation in the same way as another dream might be. There's no distance between the dreamer and the dream. In these dreams, we walk through other dimensions of ourselves to do what we need to do for survival. During one of these kind of dreams I saw myself sleeping, saw the white kitchen clock reading my time to get up, so I walked over and shook myself awake by the shoulder. I was very awake for two days after that and felt I'd learned something, though I couldn't say exactly what. I came together from two worlds, and was very happy and satisfied with life.

I think the hardest thing to deal with is a bad dream that approaches this level of dreaming. All the layers of dreaming, of which there are a great many, pass through each other, overlapping colors, scenes, and feelings, and when a nightmare touches into the real-life dream, it can be tough to get out of, like reality itself is shifting suddenly in the worst direction it can go. The love you had believed in for so long could threaten to vanish in a moment and turn into something else that betrays all your dreams.

In these times I must be very careful to allow the experience without stopping it, running from it, or judging it or the characters in it too harshly, including myself. It has interwoven itself deeply into my everyday reality, usually because it's an intimate part of it. But it's only one side, perhaps, regardless of how complex or deep or right-on all the parts appear to be. It's a harsh walk through one side of the personality and can mean a million things. It may contain a message that needs listening to. It may be a dose of what I'll get if I don't make a run for it, or it may be the provider of a horrible conversation, like the one I had at breakfast, nothing more than a way to get me out of the house and into the snow, appreciating life.

But regardless of where it goes into my waking life, it is real, and wants to be treated as such. It's like a hungry dog, or a beggar in the street, a friend disguised to test my compassion, and I've got to keep listening to it until I hear what it's saying, over and over like somebody drumming on my chest with an insistent hard forefinger. I've got to let it be there in front of me, inside of me, all around me, wherever it wants to be, until it does what it needs to do, before it finally wanders off into the labyrinth of my subconscious, the fertile ground from which it so suddenly sprang.

## Prayer to Where Bitterness
## May Lie Unattended

*Forgive me. In my own search to be true I have not given what I could, and have become part of an unanswered question. I have left too soon for us to continue. I regret this, and ask for the softness to endure, for what worked between us to endure. I can see your face turning away, your anger, and your silence. Let this be in a long box tucked among meteors bound for somewhere else. We loved and it was no accident, and now I look at my hands and ask what to do, what I have done, and how it may change into something better between us. It is simple, among a million reasons for what once was. Please let it be free now, on your side of things.*

# Seizure

Again I see I don't really know what's going on in the body. Sure, I can see causeways and interconnecting systems, but what of the motivating forces? Three days ago, in an old schoolhouse out on the frozen fields of Bavaria, a friend came near death from a seizure. After the initial trauma was over and he was in bed that night, I looked at his body in the near darkness. I felt compelled to hold my hand at the top of his head, where I saw a constriction in the glow that surrounded him. The next morning he told me he had contracted an illness as a child that left scar tissue on his brain, causing the seizures. He couldn't say anything about the mechanics of it beyond that.

Although he had gone ten years without medication, he said he was intending to start again, because the frequency of seizures had increased dramatically, and he was afraid. I agreed with him. The night before I had been alarmed by his blue color and the degree to which he was vacant, but was encouraged by his resilience in coming back.

During the night I tried generating some motion into his exhausted body, by connecting points here and there, loosening tense muscles, letting him sleep. I listened a lot, asking to know about something new to me. I knew without question it was a physical problem, one of mechanics, yet was closely interwoven with his psyche, his life situation, with all the parts of his life. But what I saw most clearly was a disfunctioning nervous system, so I began to attempt to transfer my nervous system to him. This was strictly because I didn't know what else to do. He was resting quietly, and I had seen a progression in his release of fear, and I wanted to do everything I could at a crucial time. I felt him to be a good person, so I was not afraid of getting close. I prayed for a transfer of what worked, of strength, of what I could provide him, and I prayed for a long time.

At a particular moment when I felt strongly bonded to him, my hand above his sleeping head, he awoke, looked me right in the eye with a big smile and said "Hello. How are you?" in uncharacteristically perfect English. I answered, and asked him the same question. He paused, still smiling, said "Very well," again in perfect English, and fell back to sleep immediately. Something had occurred, something subtle and hard to accurately define, a drop into another level of being.

The next morning he looked strong, happy, and fairly free, and he told me he'd never felt this way after a seizure. I took a long walk in the woods and drew a picture of him in the pine needles, letting the picture draw itself. It came out of a deep need for me to see all of this in another way. The picture had a lake at his feet, with fingers of water reaching down into the soil, with him standing in it. It had a line surrounding his whole body, inches away from the surface. Long lines came down from the space around the drawing to touch the line around his head, around the crown, like a radiance. Other lines running parallel to the surrounding line buoyed his shoulders, and others joined his knees to the earth.

This picture, in a private glade, was a drawing of his condition and his cure, and came from deep in me, yet was very simple, childlike and primitive. When I told him about it he smiled a lot, sobered, and smiled again with recognition. It worked. We agreed this drawing would collect strength in the woods there, and would continue to serve him. We agreed he could use my nervous system as long as he needed it without a loss to me, and in fact, with a gain, like having a blood-brother.

All this is a long way from scar tissue and medication, in some ways of seeing the body, but does not run contradictory. In the same way one sense grows when another is stifled or broken, the agreement in vision between my friend and me compensates for the inability of energy to pass through the scar tissue. The electro-magnetic field that surrounds the body is part of the nervous system, so our holding a common vision of this area actively enters the nervous system through the imagination, another part of the nervous system. Perhaps the immediate physical stricture can be aided by a "non-physical" passageway being opened in a mind long preoccupied with the physical and emotional problem. He has been "releasing" for many years, but not generating compensatory passageways for the release.

Some might say this is the meeting of the physical with the metaphysical, and perhaps it is, but to me it's little more than a deep desire to find another tool among many, to find a solution. I told my friend I agreed with his need for medication, with a trusted doctor, to find a balance, stability, and predictability in which he can build strength and endurance.

I keep seeing things this way all the time, that all the sources need to be used to gain strength and confidence, and there is no argument between the metaphysical and physical, between psychology, medicine, and faith healing, as far as I'm concerned. It's a question of application, function and integrity. We understand little of how it all works, but we know the body heals itself, and sometimes the more we do to fix it the more problems and dependencies we create, and this is true in all branches of healing, from conventional medicine to the psychic.

I am completely set down by all of this, by the body itself, the mind, the confidence my friend put in our vision, the results of this confidence, and by the vision itself as it springs into view. The knowledge and skill of modern medicine equally amazes me and I respect it tremendously, regardless of the arrogance of so many physicians that their knowledge is definitive. But alternative healers are equally as myopic and bigoted.

For me again, what I do is to watch, listen, and say what I see, and I don't really know a damned thing. I was scared that night with my friend, really scared. How the things happen that do I'll probably never know, but only be able to have a few guesses at. I feel grateful in my bones about it, that it helps sometimes, but I recognize without any doubt that it only happens between certain people and that outcome is never predictable. It's a sometimes blessing, and nothing more, nothing to chase down and capture. I keep saying this to myself. It's easy sometimes, hard sometimes, and sometimes impossible to talk about.

I feel very small thinking about all of this tonight. Outside, the winter night is fixing to teach us the meaning of cold, and tears are welling up inside of me. Somewhere out there my friend is riding the night train to Paris.

# Song Prayer

*Bring me the right song, the one that comes from everywhere at once, giving birth to me, the one that reaches fingers into the sky around me, the one that hears the murmuring quail and the hawk's call, the distant rustle of the sea. Bring me the one that hears her heart calling from inside of me, the one that comes with no boundaries, that divides nothing from inside of me, but that fills me with this living, the one that listens softly as it sings to me.*

# Crystal Power

I was in a basement in the Austrian Alps, a room full with the mouths of crystals. They were my birthstones, blistering purple amethyst jaws open in memory of being stolen from the earth. Some of them were huge, two and three feet tall, but they lay still, cut in half by rude electric knives that exposed their inner workings to the eyes of those seeking their power. A man lay on the floor before me, my hands gently rocking him back and forth, shaking his muscles and bones loose, connecting old wounds with new circuitry, new possibilities, crossing the boundaries of scars with potential, extending the viscera into the electric air. It was a disturbing of long held patterns, a reaching into still flesh and muted colors to excite the brilliance that struggled toward the surface, the brightness that shone in his eyes when he spoke of what he knew, the stars, the long sleep of Jupiter, the tenderness of the moon. There was a coolness on his skin, an aggregation of years, a stasis gathered in the legs, on the neck, between the shoulders, a pale green doldrum of stasis that kept crying out from behind a locked door, a huge old wooden door made long ago. We rocked against the door, beseeching quietly, steadily, for the change that waited beneath. I hummed to myself and worked the flesh, brought the bread into the texture needed, felt the electricity rise into the chimera, and kept moving forward.

Then suddenly, without warning, a swirl of darkness came up around me, and I was swept into nausea and a cold sweat. I looked at my hands and saw that nothing came up into me through them, nothing racing up the veins or along the surface of the skin like snakes into my brain, nothing alien from him to me. All was intact, and we were separate in our joining, yet a powerful force was alive in the room that threatened to deal me a blow. I felt no malevolence, yet my balance was quickly going, so I narrowed my eyes, concentrated on my solar plexus and waited, still moving slowly. A great rush of air spun up around my shoulders, surrounding us both, then lifted away out of the room through the open windows. I could see nothing, but something had gone. I felt the presence of the crystals, and an emptiness that now pervaded them. The spirit of them had left, their essence, to find its place back in the earth. A great wailing came to me then, a deep sorrow of stone having been cut, a pain in the earth where the magic no longer lay, and a searching was begun then, as birds might seek last year's nest over hundreds of miles. It was a migration toward balance, of magnetism, a central balance in the land someone had stolen and sold. I felt the ancestors in my heart praying forgiveness, and in the room a lightness began surrounding us as the power had before, and the man's body changed into something lighter, his nerves reaching into the space around him with new eyes, looking here and there with curiosity, trepidation, and excitement. He would call it a new dimension.

Weeks later I climbed a tower in Vienna, and from the top I looked in the four directions. The sun was setting in what appeared to be the east, and I wondered if that could be so in this crazy world. It took me some time to establish my position in the center, and I realized with a surprise that ever since that time in the room with the crystals, I had not known the four directions. I had been without the most basic orientation I know, and as I listened to this news I heard the crystals lamenting, searching for their homes too, somewhere out in all that space. I saw them spinning here and there, traveling over continents in a moment, passing over their homes unknowingly in confusion. Yet they were on their journey, free and wild, uncontained, finally. They had escaped, and when they left a part of me went with them, a simple, elemental part of me that knew where they belonged. They had been imprisoned in one spot, sought for power and knowledge, elements of a deep curiosity at the workings of nature. I wanted to take them into the forest and bury them, to cover them with cool damp earth the way I might cover my sleeping lover with a blanket and a kiss of deep melancholy.

All this was very strange to me, although understandable. Many of the difficult events of those weeks came under a different light, and a great blending of irony and delicacy and humor filled me. I marveled that although I had not even known where the sun rose and set, I had seen it. I had lived even in this time, as though in a cocoon of new space, unknowing that it was new space, totally ignorant of my lack of orientation, and I had survived and prospered. Beneath even the most basic senses of balance another layer of fitness had been exposed to me. The gods fairly chortled to me, and I finally had to tilt my head back in a great peal of belly laughter that still reverberates through my skull. I saw the weaknesses of that time, the meanderings, the turnings in the night, and felt the protection of my deepest emerging senses in the strange face of chaos. I felt I could go almost anywhere in this manner of faith. It sat me down into a quiet prayer.

# Obligation Prayer

*May I keep my spirit free, that I might always know the obligations of love, the need to further, to be unafraid in the face of Power, no matter what appearance it may take. Give me strength to see the needs around me, and to make the choices that build lives. Let me stay true to my word, and to your desire, and let me not feed blindness or greed. Let me feel the truth even from where I don't know, and let my love be always where it comes back real. Let me weave through false beauty to the center of the world intact. Because I owe you this much, so may it come to pass, soon.*

## Saturday Munich

Everything is white outside the car. Three old people stand talking in the cold, their bodies hunched over. They punctuate sentences by leaning forward toward each other, like birds in the snow, winter feathers puffed out. They part with gestures of affection, and the man among them walks by where I sit, his face falling into hard lines like stone, as his friends disappear into whiteness, tree branches reaching white into the sky, wooden fences and old concrete buildings tipped with snow. His face is red in all this white. I think it's time for me to go home to wait for the yellow acacia, and to call my father on the telephone.

## Prayer for Completion

*Resolution wants to come around, like a hungry cat. Let this be. Obfuscations swim between us like dark walls that threaten to live forever. Let them turn to mist, that we might see the eyes staring from the other side, hopeful. Two arms open to the sky to ask you in, love. Please come this way, and grasp the future in your own strong hands. Deliver it to our feet, and to our hearts, in a way we can't deny. Let it come all the way around, always.*

# Meeting a Baby

I have just touched elation, and everything is welling up in my throat. It's so dark outside, despite the moon, and the stars nestled in her presence like gathered children, that I hunker myself into a fetal embrace, waiting. I close my eyes, listening. I begin to ask for all my desires, to feel those who love me calling in the night. Over and over they call my name, calling just for the sound of being heard, like coyotes in a frenzy of song, like blue-jays in a flurry of sound. I bend my neck, bow my head from side to side, scratch my eye and listen. There was a man today who asked me a thousand questions to alleviate his hesitations, to touch his fears, to rest a hand against malaise and fill it with purpose. But I could do nothing to answer him. My own history has filled to overflowing with despair, and I have turned circles in dark corners for centuries like a dog searching for the right spot to lie down. I saw an intrepid spirit in the man, a glow of humor sprung from sadness, the tear in the clown's eye, and I fixed my gaze there for over an hour and knew that I could not let that vision go, for fear that we both might spin off into an endless blue universe alone. We were talking about our work here, and he mentioned suicide several times.

Coming back from Germany on the jet wind, I sat next to a nine week old baby. She stared into my eyes for a long while, and I told her in English how beautiful I thought she was, that her eyes were beautiful, her cheeks, and her lips. She looked at me without expression, focussing her entirety onto me in what looked like a huge question, an amazing expectation. Then we began to melt together, she and I, and a great love filled us both at the same time, walking us into another dimension quietly, unexpectedly. I stopped talking and gazed, filling with her, her filling with me, the steady wind blowing by our ears just outside the window. Below, the ice-caps of Greenland were glazed by brilliant clouds that threw sunlight back up against the undersides of our wings. A smile grabbed me from the middle of my heart, and my mind filled with all the experiences of my life, while the baby stared, expressionless. Then words came. "Welcome to this life," I said, glad to have such a clear spirit along. Her face exploded in a smile that included all of her, and her body twisted with the joy of it, unable to contain it. I saw my grandmother's sparkling eyes, and the baby's life passed before me, and my own as well. I saw my place with her, the stranger and the friend, and I felt the bond make something eternal between us, how she built me, how I built her, how we exploded together, clear through both our bodies.

This day will always live with me, and I felt that if I had died in the following moments, my life would have been complete, a feeling I have longed for all of my life, a feeling that is a longer growing moment gradually filling with breath and a comforting satisfaction. I wondered how it would live inside of her, if it would be with her for the rest of her life, if she would remember it one day when it was sorely needed. She went back to sleep, and I leaned back in my seat to listen to the wind and let the bright sky enter through my eyelids. I wondered if a stranger had welcomed me when I was nine weeks old, and thinking about it washed me clear through with an easy kind of gratitude.

# Home Prayer

*I am back among those who buoy me, all these birds circling, and the wind in the eucalyptus, the frogs singing all around me at night, and unspeakable joy fills me. At the ocean, dolphins come to spin circles in the waves, following me on a long walk, and the water is brisk, filling my blood with electricity. Evening gives me gold to feel, and I shake my head, kissing the ground. I am born of this land and these animals, and they have given me life over and over again. My blood comes up out of this ground, and there is nowhere else that I am given so much life. Today I thank each being that comes my way, holding me in this movement that is home, lining the avenues to my family. The world is grand, but it begins and ends here, like my life, and it is here, where the lizards come to greet me, that I am truly free. I bow my head to all who give me this, and seek to live within their will.*

# Loneliness

Is this loneliness? Or is it just that I know what I want? Yes, I want her arms around me for as many nights as I can count. I want romance of tall ships and full sails, warm winds moving us through a dream. I want to stop on an island for a millennium to gaze into her eyes, to listen to the sounds of her sleep, to feel the movement of her dreaming body.

This is longing, a mesmerization that allows me to accept the loneliness that is everywhere. The tall ship delivers me from this painful world into another, where things are seen for what they are, and tears are allowed to change the shape of separation into something better. It is everywhere, and when I move, when I breathe, eat, sleep, laugh, and play I see this loneliness bending the people to their knees.

There is a place in the city, down on the flats near the bay, where people dance below a huge screen showing gyrating figures made of two-dimensional dots, a grainy superimposition on the spirit. Four women dance together on four corners of a square, without looking at each other. One, very beautiful, wears the fashion required, long legs bared, sheathed in sheer nylon, tall heels thrusting her buttocks upward, an illusion of accessibility. She turns in rhythm, spiraling below the grinding images on the screen. She is a princess stolen from her castle by our time, by commercials and promises, rules that crushed her knowing down into hope. She dances alone, and all the princes stand before mirrors and flashing lights preening, combing their hair. The music is a combination of the sounds of baseball games and music machines, a dissonant syncopation propelling her into a nightmare of beauty, where she is a twirling piece of flesh on a wire dangling over the inevitability of aging. What will she see in her mirror when she is seventy-five?

Outside, there is an orange glow over the city, as though it were burning somewhere. It's the future, hovering over the present. It's the other side of the coin lighting our way through the parking lot. It is painfully obvious that there is much work to be done, and we stare at the sky as we walk.

When I feel this kind of aloneness I seek abstraction for solace, knowing that eventually we may all leave this planet, if not by choice, then by procrastination, all the sad faces pulling us over into an abyss, regardless of how hard we try. We are a people, and as we are instruments of time there appears to be no escape. The Hopi say the faithful will be lifted away. I wonder if the ascendance is now. And if so, what is the faith that provides? Is it a reconnection that we're addressing here? And if so, then with whom, and with what? With each other? With God? With the earth? With the water from which we came?

There are many messengers, some dancing on the parquet floor below gyrating sex symbols, some slowly circling in the sky, some looking at the lights of island cities from an eye raised only inches from the water, a wet breathing issuing forth into the night, an explosion of life in the midst of a quiet sea. I feel them all as though I live inside their lives, and this builds two hands that separate me in the center of my breast, hands that slowly and steadily pull me apart to where my heart is visible, pumping exposed to daylight and starlight, cool breezes reaching around behind it, deep into the cavity of my chest. A memory floods me, of always having been like this, and a comfort is found in the knowledge that it may never change. My body is a cape over my heart, and I hurry through the rain, bent over racing toward the dawn I see reddening the horizon. In this there is little time for loneliness, but only the necessity to arrive in time.

Meanwhile, on the deck of my ship a beautiful woman lets her hair down slowly, looking into my eyes. She is full with love and sadness, and she is unafraid to see where we are going. She tells me that the moment in which we love is huge, grander than all the destruction, yet she knows what she sees. I know too, and we don't speak of it, as though there is not enough time. We hold our people in our hands; we touch memories together and watch. Silence surrounds us in the wind and we are born into each other's body. Somehow we become the world and everything starts over again with the ability to prevail over all the gloom. Our loneliness finds a home and our fears become the song of our death, seen through a quiet eye that floats across the world no longer separate.

In this joining I accept all that I am brought to live and know, and the alienation of our time is a great sorrow, a deepening spiral in the middle of a red ocean that must seemingly always exist somewhere, one step off the edges of my being, just a heartbeat away, where I myself easily become the dancer on the hot parquet floor, spinning around inside the walls of my own invisible prison.

## Prayer to Reach You at a Distance

*My sister, these desires become a hand to cover the distance between us, both in time, and across the world. I see you always when I stare at clouds, feeling words form out of invisible sound. It is too far sometimes, like now, so I gather beaks and eyes, furs in the winter snow, sparkling light off icy branches, a rolling surf, spray racing off the wave crests like a horse's mane, and I thrust them into the sky with all my love. There must be a way to reach you. Hear me now, and fall into what we need for strength. Build with me what we need to know. Reach to me here where I stretch in hunger to feel your presence. I am waiting now. Please hear me calling. I am halfway to the moon, calling you.*

# The Vanishing Nature
# of Revelation

Ideas come and go sometimes so quick and profound, that I feel I'll never see them again. They just disappear into the evening sky, into the purple orange sky, leaving me standing feeling like a fool for not being able to hang onto them. Sometimes they're revelations, things that swell up from the depths of me, and I see my life in a beautiful clear light like it's all been given to me, and I know everything just for a few seconds. I'll stop what I'm doing and stare, maybe, awestruck that it could be so simple. I know that I'll be able to retain the vision long enough to write it down and thereby never lose it. I'm right in the middle of it. How could I ever forget? Everything makes sense, and I accept it so deeply that I must take it for granted, because then I seem to wake up out of this clarity, or go to sleep out of it; I'm not sure which is right, or the best way to see it, but I wake up suddenly realizing that it's gone, and I don't understand anything anymore, and nothing makes the same kind of sense. I may see my life all right, and have some distant kind of purpose and all, but something is missing. I don't feel in the center of it anymore, but out on the edge of it, just out of touch with the essence.

I can't figure this out, how something can come and go so fast. It's like love; not to be understood, but only known. You're either in love or you're not, it seems. If you have to think about it, chances are you aren't.

The funny thing is that I can still remember so many of these occurrences of revelation, or at least part of them. I see myself now, thinking back on it, standing in the twilight, the moon starting up behind the eucalyptus leaves, all caught up in the glow of the night sky, seeing everything crystal clear. I'm looking down at my boots, which barely shine back at me from the ground, and I feel the gravel under my feet. I see myself standing there as though it were in the future, pondering, trying to remember. It's a double twist in time, like a diver might perform into a clear blue pool. I'm up there in the future, right here in the moment, and back there in the past all at once, standing in the same position with my feet crossed, breathing and staring down-wards. I can smell the trees. I can taste the moment, but I can't tell you what my great revelation is if my life were to depend on it.

So what do I do with this slippery quality of enlightenment? I guess I get used to it, and make some axioms about nothing being forever anyhow, so I can sleep at night without thinking I'm losing my mind. The way it gives me finally is to keep listening, moving on in the trusting that it'll come again of its own accord, most likely when I quit looking for it.

It's like today I was working on a woman's body and I saw these jagged shards of electricity that looked like lightning bolts all squashed down into a drawing, like a cartoon. The woman has bad hearing, and I was trying to open up the channels so she could hear better, feel a bit better balanced and more in tune with the world around her. I had my fingers around her ears, the fingertips pressing into her skull some, feeling electric, like you do when you scuffle across the carpet, and I saw the electric lines coming around in a semi-circle wanting to connect her eyes and her ears. At first I thought it was something in my eye, so I paid it little mind, but it kept on being there, and the more I stayed with the feelings on the woman's head and in my fingers, and kept praying for her hearing and her balance, the more I saw the electricity. It had blues and golds and reds in it like a diamond does on the edges, in the center, but not somewhere you could capture it at all. It was fluid, yet maintained its shape and kept growing, as though it would surround her whole head. I thought about how people seem to want to see auras and things to understand more about life, but when I saw this I knew less. It always turns out that seeing more is knowing less. At least less of the why of it all. I might see how things come to be, or what they do, or what they look like, but why they come up out of not being there is a mystery to me.

The persistence of the sight of these electric shards settled me down some, and I began to think alongside of my seeing, and to see more alongside of the thinking. Everything grew all at once, and I felt in the center of everything, not knowing much but that I was on one end of something good, and something strong. I held to it with delicacy, softly and slowly, kept seeing the little lightning bolts, letting them be there without explanation, and they expanded out finally into a field of faint but brilliant light around her head. Some of it went into her, some went out into the atmosphere, but all of it made sense. It came and went, and while it was there it seemed to plant some seeds, because when the woman woke up she was soft and quiet, and I didn't have to shout to be heard.

Somehow there's a similarity in these two things I'm talking about, about how I lose my brilliant visions, and about how the magic comes and goes. I see a lot of people trying to grasp these things like they're cars or pretty women, trying to hold onto them and call them abilities. Some even try to teach these things, how to see them, and how to hold on to revelation. And though I'm sure some people can hold on to most anything for a long while, and squeeze every last morsel out of something, still it's all the same. When it's gone, it's gone, and all you have is the tracks of where it went. The fact that it comes is what we ought to better use our time looking at. That it comes at all, that it exists and comes to us. This is surely a good thing, and we ought to pay it its due.

I realized tonight, walking up the trail to the mailbox, that I need to be heading into the wilderness again soon. All these thoughts get me caught up too much in Mankind, in all the ways we see the workings of nature and call it our accomplishment. It gets real tiresome sometimes, how everybody goes on and on about knowledge and love and understanding. It seems to me the best way to partake of the most is to sit back with your eyes open, with your heart on clear intentions, wishing the best for the next person. It's then all the gods come quietly into the garden, making themselves known in private ways only each of us knows alone.

## Mountain Traveler's Prayer

*May you walk with eyes open into the wilderness. May the guardians walk with you, touching the skin you know, filling the air around you with strength and beauty. With each step may they be with you, and may you remember what is behind you, and feel what is to come. May your smile spread from Then to Now, and to Then again, there in the future. And may your eyes move through time like rivers beneath the eagle's gaze. May this be so, and may your feet touch the center of the earth in strength and gentleness each time. May your solitude be quiet, easy in the night, easy in the storm, easy in the crowd, and may your joining be of the right way always, where your heart finds peace. May this be so, and may we all circle in this joining to let this be. May the soft eye of the morning wolf be with you, and the magic of the jumping fish, the warm coat of the marmoset, the wisdom of the soaring golden bird, the steadiness of the falling water. May all these things be with you, inside of you, around you. May this be so. May we let this be so in this time, as our hands make a surrounding circle and touch the earth's skin. For this we give thanks, and remain in the wisdom of your way.*

# A Quick Beginning

When I first saw her I felt I could help her, that we could make the connection needed to mend her heart. It was apparent in her skin tone that she had been in pain for a long while, running at a pace not her own. The hunger walked all over her skin and through her eyes. There are many ways to see it.

Today we talked about her history briefly, and I connected with her body for a short while, going straight to loosening everything around the area of the heart, then expanding out to the limbs. She just wanted to know it's okay.

It's wonderful when it happens quickly like this. I am certain that our connection will make a huge difference for us both, infusing faith. She cried a number of times, on the wet edges of tears, seemingly of gratitude, yet not tumbling over into the weeping stages. That will come later tonight perhaps, when she is alone in bed, or driving in her car. Then she will laugh. She is a fine woman still chasing down the marriage pattern, only just beginning to become aware that perhaps the gods have something different in store for her, at least for awhile.

It occurs to me again that much of illness, heart-sickness and debilitations of the blood system and nervous system comes from a fighting spirit still searching for the proper battle to wage. Anger spinning aimlessly always surfaces in the blood, and as the heart is filled with blood, the pain may be felt in this essential passageway, this collection. This is not to over-simplify, as it's certainly not a simple occurrence. It is deeply complex, tying in to a million things around family, heritage, genetics, diet, the entire gamut. What I am saying is that there is an approach to dealing with it that is simple, and that though it is simple, it may not be easy. Again, it takes a willingness to acquiesce to something larger than oneself to utilize this view, and this is not always easily done. There are a thousand programs screaming to be heard.

Today we determined that fire was needed, and we both entered the afternoon with the desire to make fire, and to let it burn where it wanted and needed to be. This was in the heart, and in the blood. Now she won't have to do the work alone anymore; the fire will burn of its own accord. This is the surrender, and it always seems to take much time in suffering to be willing to accept this manner of being. There is great relief in this, to be sure, and it is always a great pleasure to me to find this willingness. And I begin to see that this is the place where my work lies. We can speak to the creatures inhabiting the body without fear of being ridiculous, because we know they hear. They are creatures like us, who ultimately want to live and thrive. A parasite may be spoken to and convinced that there is a better host. It's not always easy, but it is real. There are many kinds of conversations, and all living beings know the nature of relationship and communication, though the condition of our world would not make this seem to be the case.

It is a soft prayer for her tonight that courses through me. I forgot to ask her to call me to check in. I'll want to know how she is doing tomorrow. She needs protection in confidence, and may need some help with this for awhile. But ultimately she will be scintillating, as she is powerful and beautiful, a very present person with a deep passion and much to give. Perhaps her emptiness will come to its vast potential soon, and then she will begin to fill with life as never before. In this she will light up the sky, and I know this will be. It has already begun. I stand aside and watch as the future begins to burn. I felt it in her body today, and saw it in her tear-filled bright eyes.

## Prayer for Healing

*Let me not get strung out on all this magic, all this truth that is falling around me like a beautiful rain. It is softer and easier as it goes, something bright, light, touching down on the ground. Let it continue to be in this way, and when it is too heavy to stand, let me continue to stand in the confidence of benevolence. Let me always know the sources of this work, and let me never call it my own. The temptations are great, as I hear they have always been, and as my life will attest. Let me not forget this. Four winds, blow me this way and that to make me always know how small I am in your eyes, and continue to tender me your magic breath. All this wonder breaks open every day to reveal more and more, and a deep power emerges all around me, something like a huge storm brewing, then taking shape. Let me stay quiet in this rain, holding my palms to the sky gratefully, knowing the days to come, the times to come, the swing of the pendulum. Let me be ready, and let me stay in your grace. It is here that everything matters, and it is here that nothing changes to destruction. This is what must be. Let me be in this way with you.*

# Concepts in Healing

It's funny how the ego goes. When I try to describe the healing work to someone it gets removed a step or two, and my sense of myself as a 'healer' begins to come through. Then when I begin to work again, I have to spend time getting through this image and the techniques that I've described. I worked on a number of people in Europe, with strong results, and afterwards answered their questions about energy fields, meditations, and what I saw. I felt the healings taken in as lessons and teachings, and when this happened much of the essence began to fade away. In this conceptual process part of the magic of the joining disappears. The love gets buried too easily in notions of auras, subtle bodies and etheric bodies. These aspects may be true, but they're far less than what's really going on. They are another form of the same control that causes the problem in the first place.

Why do we want to hold the magic at a distance, or to own it, to contain it, to call it something? Isn't the immersion enough? I think it's so strong and so subtle at the same time, so intimate and revealing, that it needs to be objectified for some kind of protection of the status quo. When this happens I can see the thought processes beginning to obscure many of the connections. The man who is cruel may continue to be cruel, to call his newfound sensitivities his own, and to miss how sensitivities must be measured in their depth and effectiveness on those around him. They must be measured not by his own freedoms, but by the obvious freedoms of those he has been controlling, and he must be willing to surrender his own knowledge to perceive the knowledge of others, the knowledge they might have of him, and to listen to what they are saying. But something may be deeply broken. He might be afraid to care, it seems, or he might be listening to a voice that places him a step ahead of others. In his mind and motives he might be an oriental king walking ten steps ahead of the woman, in spirituality, in evolution. It's a fantasy, as all dominant male styles finally are, and it's easy to say those beneath him must learn strength. "Yes, she's getting there. It's very good," he might say, smiling without seeing his part in the pain, simply because he doesn't want to. Active choice is a true dynamic here, regardless of the effects of personal history, and cultural blindness validates tons of shit. For instance, how long has it been woman's job to live the suffering of the man?

Today I worked on an old friend, connecting points here and there, to the tune of much moaning in pleasure. She was vocal throughout the time I was touching her, telling me what she felt. I worked on connecting opposite sides of her body, but off-center, like a counter-point most of the time, searching for the spots that would give a little, receive the touch a bit deeper. The moans were predictable. It was subtle, and very strong. When this way comes through I feel the touches to be time capsules, seeds of love and connection I know will come through in the days to come. We had talked about structure and definition the night before, and how easily these things limit the experience.

Afterwards we were sitting on her front porch, under the walnut tree and passion-flower vine, and she began to rub my neck. I moaned. It felt fantastic, and I was sorely needing this depth of touch. She went on and on, trying this and that, getting deeper and deeper. It kept getting better, and soon I realized I was getting some of the best body work I'd ever had. At one point she put her head against the center of my back and pushed, butting like a goat. She said "I see antlers. Elk antlers."

I laughed and asked her what she meant, joking, and she said, "I don't know. I just see antlers," in a dramatic voice. So it was antler technique she was doing, we agreed, which quickly ran through many plays on words to become Elken Technico, an esoteric workshop offered for only six hundred dollars per day. We kept laughing, and she kept working on me. Soon I was putty in the sun, moaning and laughing, and new pictures of my body were popping into my mind by the second. Our conversations about technique and description kept coming back over and over, and I could only chuckle deep inside. She seemed amazed at my profound experience. She was just paying me back, she said. It was plain and simple to her.

All this was a big circle, and this is really how it works. I don't blame people for walking out on this world, on the action, the money-making and the politics and the education. It seems like every time something good comes along it no sooner gets born than it's sucked up into the machine, processed and sold, or some church is formed around it. It's undoubtedly a crazy world, and two friends taking care of each other on a sunny day is the highest art there is, I'm convinced. We didn't sell each other tickets, and if we're lucky we won't remember what happened long enough to prevent it from happening by surprise once again.

I keep finding the precious in the simple, and in this I am again and again laid back against the truth of what I don't know, and what it seems I never can know. From here I keep starting out from scratch, and I'm just now beginning to see this is the very best place to both begin and end.

# Sun Prayer

*Come right inside of me now, clear through my blood, through my lungs, into my chest, deep and moving. Fly through me warm like fire, and touch my knowing with your dispassionate life. Don't stop anywhere I might reflect on what you are, pondering on intricate meanings, but course through me like water running down a mountain, free as you need to be. I will give you my body this way, and surrender to your need in me. Come down across the world to touch me now. I am ready.*

# Instant Healing

Something new has transpired. I see now that healing can be complete in one period of time, suddenly, perhaps instantaneously. All the patterns are there, and the light may pass through all of them at once, all the passageways, into a new-old way of being. This is nothing about somewhere else, or something else, something removed or alien, but is more a returning, and may be gentle, pervasive, and almost imperceptible. Sometimes it can only be seen in what life begins to offer. As I see this I'm drawn to move directly into it, to penetrate deeply for a moment, like diving into a huge pool. It's vast for a second, connected everywhere perhaps. I can't tell, but it feels so. There is nothing left out, no dark places, yet not everything is apparent, and there's no need for it to be. Again, it's a joining, without the need for it to be on any linear process, a function of time, or a long road.

It's the bath. It's the darkness where color is born, where shape begins, and where we inhabit the body in peace. The peace is the key. It's the impetus, and it emerges more each day, expansive, infinite, everywhere at once.

I saw this yesterday, standing in the sun under the pear tree, and how it moves quickly through space to someone else. It's more of an internal sense of completion, and it may come and go. It fits with "working" from a distance, a function of prayer. Tonight I felt it in someone's chest, as my fingers went deeper and deeper, not so much into the flesh, but into the body in another sense, as the whole of what we live inside of, around and through.

This makes each time full with potential and infinitely interesting. I begin to wonder what limits healing then. Is it conceptual notions of the body? Just going back to what it was? No, because that movement is fine too. Maybe it's not seeing the essence, and we get dragged back into the periphery. Or maybe we just lose focus. That's an important one, easy to do and inevitable.

But all this is beginning to meander. I just wanted to say what I saw, that it can be a one-shot deal. It's an awesome thing to see and begin to touch, yet simple as a baby's smile. Yes, that's where it is, in the center of that smile and newness and trust and unknowing. There's a ton of Zen words for it, but it's just a flicker of firelight in the night, the lick of a flame that never quits, but keeps on illuminating from the center out. It's another step, a quiet one wrapped around an acquiescent soul.

# Something Big

There's something huge moving around in the universe, something undefined and portentous, like a big hand forming that might pick us all up and throw us across time like a scattering of seeds. Or like an eye forming out of darkness, not in judgment or any kind of distant evaluation or distant presence, nothing to seek or look toward, but something incredibly present and causal, almost as though it binds us together in some way we can't touch, but only know. And although there is the sense of a constant presence already, to be sure, this something big is like a storm. It's a form of change in light, like at dawn or dusk. It's a voicing of what we know, something painful yet not stuck there, moving outward into joy as well, and even beyond this polarity. It's nothing other-dimensional, but more a settling in to what already exists. I'm reaching toward it with these words that feel like early raindrops from its coming, the first sounds pattering on the roof. I want to say it's good, but can't. I want to say it's new, but it isn't. It seems I can only sit in silence with my brow scrunched up listening to it roll on under us, over us, all around us. I shake my head from side to side, looking, listening, waiting for what keeps telling me with great insistence that it's already here.

# What Do We Know
# About the Ancestors?

Listen. There's a rolling rhythm from outside. Crickets. It's like this with the old ones, isn't it, how they sing to us from the inside so deeply we call it something else, say it's coming from another world, another place. We fantasize them and make churches in the mind, while they scowl and laugh and cajole us with songs we know as our own.

I have a sister in Tasmania. She loves me on the inside, and calls me a blessing, and I hear her voice inside of me laughing, crying, complaining, moaning and bitching, then softening into the truth she knows so well, where we stand in the same blood and look into the sky together. I can only say a few words about this because just before we said good-bye on the phone everything flew between us like a scattering of quail into bright light, essential, brilliant, beautiful and full. I see her swimming in the river beneath giant cottonwoods, under the wings of the ancient huge grey river birds. I smile to think of her, and I fill to feel her, listen to her voice, to her ears, and I remember all the silences we have found surrounding us in great peace. We have been found building something in the sand, oblivious to the darker natures of the world, insistent, reaching, with wise old eyes in the faces of children. Who can live without such connections?

Oh my sister I have bowed my head so many times to find you this year, swirling in a dark anger in my soul, terrified of the usury, imprisoned in the fear it could never change, that images of the new world to come were nothing more than huge machines of oppression, black magic dressed as God. In the middle of this I have laid on my back in the rain, my skin against cool stones at the top of a giant waterfall, listening to the roar and the singing of the water. All around me clouds rose from the bases of trees to rise into the arms of the sky's clouds, waiting, and waterfalls poured from everywhere to make the river beside me, and I could hear nothing separate from anything else. In this place you came to join me, and when I felt your presence I was glad, but still no smile crossed my face. The trees stood dark green and pungent in the rain, and there was something deep to enter for us all. A young woman lay beside me in desperation, confusion too permanent a state of mind to see beyond, even survival forgotten. I picked a small stone from the water and held it to the sky and asked for a gathering. You came closer, and you brought your clan with you, and before the day was over we had all seen the meeting place together. The young woman held me close to her, and I smelled her wet hair amongst the pines, and the tears streaming down her face with the rain. She laughed loud and long in her crying, and when we ran down the mountain we couldn't stop smiling.

In my silence I know what is true, what has happened in this timelessness, this precious field where we run. We call it our work, our obligation, our gift and our cross. We say a million things about it, and labels dance around our loneliness, trying to make the hard parts okay, but there is really no choice in these matters. We are found, once again, in this giving, for giving is what it is, plain and simple, the greatest gift.

## Time Prayer

*I want to stay right here, because there is nowhere else, here in this time. If I reach behind me with one hand, and before me with the other, I can touch both edges of history, like two trees in a dark night. I can tilt my head back and drink the stars, can hear the owls talking across the canyon, can watch morning come easily from the east. It is all here, as it's always been. Remind me Lord, of where I belong, and keep me here with these people, where the voices have faces and there is no emptiness that stays.*

# Who's Safe Anymore?

I just spent the evening with some wonderful people, at a sleazy bar here in town. Well, it wasn't that sleazy, but it did represent the drunken quotient around here, the glazed eyes, the macho stance, the hungry stare. I wondered how the hell anyone in this kind of stupor could get laid, and I saw it in the after-hours, the desperate fucking, trying hard to find the heart in the midst of the liquor and sadness, the removal from the reality of the genitals' connection to the soul. I remember what my ex-wife said, about how you can't make love with someone without getting close, no matter what you might think.

It wasn't that everyone was looking for sex, but many were. In the group I was in there were great talks about biases and racism and elitist thought and writing to make experience known and real, and the girl I came to see ran off in the middle of the night to get stoned with some guy I wouldn't trust to cross the street with me. Ah, she's young, and can take care of herself, I thought after she had left, but I knew better, and had to send prayers her way. Where can any of us stop working? How in the hell do you separate work from anything else? Even now, just before dawn, I bow my head and send her the love that confides, that abides and stays firm. It's such a sad and lonely place.

How can it be understood?

A young Irish-Cherokee woman and I had breakfast til four AM, sharing the same attitude, something mixed in our blood, I'd guess, the laughter, the orneriness and the earth magic, the connection. We were both worried about our mutual friend, the one who'd gone off, but we didn't talk about it, all in the name of freedom.

I was pissed. I didn't like the trade she'd made. How to deal with it tomorrow? Time and circumstance would tell the tale. The truth would come to be known, and I love this girl deep inside, and can feel her pain and confusion like it's my own. Still, in all this empathy, there's little I can do. I feel as though in some ways she's both my lover and my daughter. And the boundaries are clear between us. How can I penetrate her sadness to impart the joy that frees? And, who am I to presume so much?

So the Irish-Cherokee woman and I drank coffee and told life stories and I smiled inside to know her. If it weren't for my ears I'd lose my mind. I know only what I know, which whittles my courage down into knowing I'll get by, staying reasonably away from the predominate shit in this world, but what of a young woman like this, who sees easily as much of the shortcomings as I do, yet presses onward? I stand in awe, and still I see all the questions of the dreamer. Is this real? Will the best things come to pass?

I want to stand as guardian to these dreams, because I still believe in them too, though I am twice as old as this young woman. I see those who've cast aside the dreams, and I see pale faces deprived of magic, of the simplicity in a child's morning eye, in a child's dancing step. I refuse to introduce what the pessimist calls reality, cold hard reality, because I still refuse to believe it myself. I'm told to prepare young people for the real world, yet I see the ravages of the real world all around me, especially on the faces of those who advocate it. I won't do it, because I'd be cutting off my own face, my own deepest beliefs. Tales of warriors, chivalry, and honor still stand as sentinels inside of me, and even in the relative waning of my life I grasp romance with a firm grip. There is no better way visible, as far as I can see. In this eye a deep courage is on fire. It's something of hope, aware as a morning coyote. There is no turning away. I know it as surely as I see the goose crossing the road. Not only do I believe, but I have no doubt, and the perseverance I see around me is created by benevolent centuries, ancestors, forefathers, by the language itself, and the heart we have been given.

In this I stand listening in awe. There is no better place and I have nothing more to say but this tonight.

# Prayer of Thanks

*There's got to be a form of you tonight, Lord, because I feel you alive everywhere all around me. Many people spoke to me tonight, and there was love in all their eyes, and then the woman called me from the other side of the world and we were together for some precious minutes on the telephone. And now I sit listening to the night song outside this little bunkhouse at the top of the valley where the fog reaches to. I stood in the mist before I came inside and listened to the stars talk like crickets singing. You are with me, and I want to ask you for everything, for money, and for love to hold me in her arms tonight, but you tell me to be patient, to wait for the right time for both, and so I do, and then you hand me a face of courage, seen in all those around me dealing with their own suffering, dancing 'til midnight like brothers and sisters, raising their arms to the sky, rolling into the river of humanity on a steady rhythm that seems to keep coming and coming.*

*I will sleep in your arms tonight, and if I ask for more than you have given me, forgive me, and listen to my plea. It's an easy one, and is only for the icing on the cake. You have given it all to me in these years, and you continue to look deep inside me as though I were the only person on earth. I thank you for this attention, and strive to live in your grace accordingly.*

# American Beauty

I met a woman today who rode her horse from Corralitos, California, to Maine. It took her three and a half years on a beautiful roan appaloosa named Rosie. I saw a picture of Rosie, who'd passed away just recently. The woman had a dog with her too, but they stole her dog somewhere in the country where little dogs were valuable for hunting birds. It was a smart dog, she said, who'd be good for hunting small animals where they needed dogs to move under low brush. She got another dog when she rode through Memphis, got him from the animal shelter, and she had to call the mayor to keep from paying the fourteen dollar fee. She'd offered to pick up the dog just before they killed it in the morning, but the lady at the shelter said they couldn't do that; that she'd have to pay the fee or they'd kill the dog. She told the lady she could afford to feed the dog, but not to buy it. She didn't believe in buying animals that needed homes anyway, so she called the mayor, who had read about her in the newspaper that morning. She was pretty well famous by then, having just ridden into

downtown Memphis on a roan appaloosa all covered with trail dust. It ain't a common sight these
days, it seems. The mayor covered everything in fif-
teen minutes, including shots, tags, collar and the
works, free of charge.

It wasn't that this woman had simply done this
trip that impressed me about her. More, it was her
attitude. She swore in just the right places, walked
with a sure step, and had a kindly eye that didn't
look away at all, except when it was just right. She
smiled a lot and shook her head when she didn't
understand some of the ways of people. She said
there were a lot of nice people out there, meaning in
the world, who were ready to sit down and bullshit
with a stranger. That's the way she said it. And she
said she tried things both ways on her trip, one day
with a wave and the next without. On the waving
days people would stop and talk to her, ask her
where in the hell she was riding that horse to anyhow, and their jaws would drop when she said to
Maine, and when she answered further that she
was coming from California, on top of that, and all
this questioning would be out in the flatlands of
Tennessee somewhere, their jaws would drop down
still another notch. On the non-waving days she
said people wouldn't talk to her much, and she said
she learned a lot from that.

She said the only problems she had were with
rangers and highway patrolmen, who'd tell her she

couldn't ride alongside the highway, or cross state park boundaries on her horse. She said one ranger asked her where she thought she was going, out in the Grand Tetons in Wyoming, and when she told him he paused a bit and asked her if she had a license. She asked him for what, of course, and he paused again and said something about a license to ride a horse across the park. She asked him what was on the other side of the park, up the road, and if she could get her horse shod there, and when he answered that she could, she told him that was where she was going. She asked him where to get the license to ride her horse across the park, and he said he didn't know. So she told him he was wasting her time and his own at the same time, bid him a good day and rode on up the road. She never saw him again, just left him standing there mumbling something about a license.

A highway patrolman in Arizona told her to get off the side of the road and when she politely told him she had the right to be there, he said she didn't. She told him to check the law, to call in, but he said he didn't have to, that he was the law. She told him he wasn't and kept on riding. Her last words to him at that point in their relationship were that if he was going to act like an asshole then she was going to treat him like one. He chased her on foot a bit, running and holding down his flapping holster, so she broke Rosie into a trot, and he had to walk back a piece to get his car. She knew he couldn't arrest her because he couldn't leave the horse and the dog alongside the highway unattended. And she knew the law. She was no dummy. She'd called and checked on the laws before she left. She kept calling him sir and telling him to call in and check the law, which he said he didn't need to do, and which he didn't do for the three whole days he tried to corral her at the offramps. She'd just ride around him and leave him flashing his lights and honking his horn and getting red in the face, waving at her alongside his squad car. At the end of the third day he apologized, since he finally did call and find she had a right to be there. They don't own the highway on forty feet of each side, she told me, and you can do whatever you want there.

She finished describing this guy by shaking her head and saying he was a real "rear end." She had a good way of putting things. When he apologized she told him he could of saved himself a lot of trouble. She said those guys were pretty much all the same, cops, and couldn't see what was real for all the rules swimming around inside their brains. She said she'd listen to anybody who was making sense, but when somebody wasn't making sense, it didn't make any sense at all to listen to them.

We talked about marriage some, and she said she was a widow, and that she'd never marry again. She said she didn't need any boss. She had a man friend there she called her little dude, saying he was a good little dude, but that she'd never marry him no matter how much you paid her. They'd been together nine years.

He was a real nice guy, with a good straight eye and a solid handshake, from Texas, who looked and sounded just like my Grandpa. I thought she was right about it all. She didn't need a boss, and they had a good respect between the two of them, it seemed to me. He was the one who showed me the picture of Rosie, with the little dog sitting high on the saddle, the woman standing grinning beside them both. He said the dog was a little boss himself who thought he was a big German shepherd trapped inside a fox terrier body, who didn't like anybody but the woman. He was a good little shit, the man said, laughing. These people knew animals.

We talked about coons, and what a nuisance they can be, how cocky and destructive they are. And about cats, how they own people, rather than the other way around. She said she always looked into an animal's eyes to tell how they were. We talked some about man's cruelty to man, and about Nazi Germany, and she said she never saw animals treat each other so bad. I agreed with her.

We talked about hunting and she said she'd hunted all across the country with a shot of whiskey. She'd soak feed in whiskey, marinate it, she said, then put it out for quail and rabbits, who would eat it to the point they'd get so drunk they couldn't run, and she'd pick them up and kill what she could eat.

I liked this woman a lot. She brought me back into knowing my roots again and again, with her accent, her swearing, her kind eyes, her love of animals, and her understanding of just about everything, even how she understood not understanding itself. She made me feel at home here in this land. When I asked her what she did all those years crossing the country she said she bullshitted with people. So that's what we did all afternoon, bullshitted and drank beer. I'd gone to look at a piece of property she was selling, her home, and got a huge dose of goodness for my trouble.

I saw Rosie's grave on the hillside, surrounded with stones, a circle of them in the center, where the heart of a laying down horse might be, flowers growing across it in the dry sandstone. She said she'd never buried a horse before, but Rosie'd been with her for thirty-one years. Rosie's leg had finally played out on her and they had to put her down. I remembered my Grandpa's old quarter horse. The woman and I had a moment of silence looking down on Rosie's grave. I wanted to buy the property just to be close to the horse who carried this wonderful woman so far across this land and so quickly into my heart.

As we were talking there was one point when she said it was time for a change, and I thought I saw a step deeper into her. She said she was out of challenge here, that everyone knew her, and that she knew everyone else. She wanted to move somewhere new, where nobody knew her and she had to go out and earn new friends. That was the word she used, earn. She said you had to keep learning, all your life, and that was what it was all about. If you couldn't do that, then what's the point, she said. There's a lot of land to see and people to meet, and she was ready to move on. As I looked into her eyes I remembered a comment she'd made about not getting attached to another horse, and I wondered if she had to leave Rosie's grave behind, if that wasn't the reason to keep moving. I don't know. I'm sentimental about these things myself, and regret I can't visit my old Indian pony's grave, the horse I grew up with. I swim in the river I grew up on sometimes, and it all comes back, washing through my mind like it was yesterday, with a great longing. This woman said she wanted a pond on some flat land, where she could raise catfish, and I remembered the catfish we lived on out on the Stanislaus River.

But it wasn't the memories she brought to mind that made me love this woman. It was just who she was, all the basic things she had that I admire in people, like defiance and courage and softness all rolled into one. Wisdom, directness, fun and humility stuck together.

She said she talked like a man because she'd learned to speak English in pool halls. She only spoke French as a child, being French-Canadian, and didn't much like to talk with women. She said they talked in circles without getting to the point, talking round and round things just pointing at them, without really saying them. I don't know about that, but I couldn't help thinking that if I was older, or she was younger, and her little dude wasn't around for her, and things were different for me, that I'd like to get to know her. She's still pretty, and has a strong body.

But the essence of the day with her was something powerful, beyond all surface things. It was her eyes, like looking into the eyes of an animal to know it, to see its character, its strengths and weaknesses. Her eyes were clear to me, like looking into a friendly desert sky, like laying on your back in the high country, looking out into heaven. I could almost hear her horse breathing next to her on a Montana plain in the middle of the night, coyote's telling of her coming far-off down the road. I went with her on that journey, riding my own wishes that I'd been there some of that time, feeling the horse move under me, looking up at a sunrise with her, or waiting for the beans and corn to heat up on a mid-day flat desert rock. Or even better, in the late evening mist, crouching around a small fire, watching the flames dance off the center of her eyes, reaching out into a vast, silent, living darkness just like the middle of creation itself, the place where all the love in this world is really born, and you know everything. You just know, and nothing else matters, but that one huge moment of watching the fire sparkle off someone's eye.

## Prayer For Accidental Meetings

*Oh yes, please keep bringing the people into my life like this, with all their courage and fire, determination and righteousness. Bring them from everywhere, when I least expect it and most need it. You take good care of me in this way. They come from everywhere, each ready to give, to meet straight on without deceit, but in the center of what's needed. This is a great blessing you keep bringing to me and I feel an endless chain of beauty waiting out there in many forms and faces. You keep delivering this to me. I thank you over and over and open my eyes into the brightness of your night sky, satisfied.*

# Spirit Dance

I went to a dance in Watsonville tonight, and there were only two or three white couples there. It was hot Mexican polka music with rock and roll flair, blaring full blast through the old veteran's hall. There were a lot of gang guys with tattoos and slicked back hair, and very good vibes. My companion and I walked around the block, through a dark alley where a bunch of guys were hanging out by an old lowered chevy, and they said hi as we walked by and greeted them, again, with good vibes.

When I was in the bathroom a guy easily twice as big as me came in to pee beside me. It was a one-trough system, without any dividers or space between, and it was small, and since both of us were kind of big we were standing very close to one another. I told him I thought the band was hot, and he nodded and kept peeing. After a silence he said, "You know, this is good," and he let the words hang in the air between us. "This is beautiful," he said, and he kept looking into my eyes. I agreed that it was beautiful. Then he said, "You know, we can do it," and again he let the words float around to become as big as he was in the air of the bathroom, his head tilted back so he was looking down at me out of the bottoms of his eyes. "It's up to us," he said, and I said, "Yeah it is. And we can do it. We gotta do it." He said "It's up to us," again, and I said "Ain't nobody else gonna do it." He stared at me, and we both kept peeing straight ahead into the trough. "We got no choice," I said, and he repeated, "It's up to us." There was another long silence between us, looking into one another's eyes, peeing straight ahead into the trough, the muffled sound of the band banging against the old plaster wall in front of us.

Then he raised his free hand to me, high in the air, about the level of his eyes, and we shook in the old brother way, holding hands for a long while, peeing straight ahead, and he said, "Thank you for understanding that," and he nodded slowly, very strong. I nodded back, and said "Thank you too." I let go of his hand then to finish peeing and zip up my pants. He was much bigger than me so he kept on peeing, and when I turned to leave we both smiled at the same time. Two other guys came into the bathroom while all this was going on, took one look at us standing there shaking hands, looking heavy into one another, and turned around to leave. The image of the two of us standing at the trough clasping our free hands, looking into each other's eyes, passed between the two of us clearly, and it was a powerful and good emotion filling that funky bathroom, something real.

Moments like this make it for me, where the comic and the real get down together and brotherhood shines through it undaunted and unembarrassed. Later on the dance floor we crashed into each other during an exuberant polka and I wondered if he had told his lady about our meeting in the bathroom. I told my partner and she cracked up laughing, then sobered and said, like he had, "It's beautiful, really beautiful, and there aren't enough times like that in our lives."

Now, I haven't shaken hands with a peeing stranger too many times myself, but I gotta say I'd gladly do it again if it was real. It was a good thing, and at the same time I'm glad there are other ways to know we're all in this mess together, and that somebody else besides me believes that we can do it. It's funny how the gods pick these places to put a bit of sanity into an overburdened world. For myself I'm not going to complain; I'm just glad they do it at all. And when I really think about it, it's actually not a bad combination to relieve the bladder and the soul at the same time. It's pretty thorough.

# Fear and Leaving

In talking with a Buddhist friend the other day about fear, I came to guess about a few things. We just leave when we get scared, is what I kept thinking. I remembered when I was in the Orient as a young man, practicing Martial Arts and Zen meditation, I'd heard a lot about getting outside the body, and I'd practice climbing inside of light bulbs and such, seeing things within things within things. I had some esoteric experiences, and still, I maintained my cool very well. I was young.

Just before I came back, after being there close to two years, I was out in the East China sea one afternoon with some guys, way out in a small rubber raft. I was diving in an area where it went from shallow to deep instantly, and you could float out over canyons that dropped down into forever, bluer and bluer off into nothingness. I saw that Zen nothingness wasn't black, but most likely a deep sea blue. I was swimming around a big piece of coral, about twelve feet under, holding my breath, when a fifteen-foot long shark came up from the nowhere to greet me. His mouth was open big enough to get my body in easily, without even scraping the double row of teeth. His eyes were at the level of my eyes, staring into me with a dull ancient quality. He was an organic eating machine without compassion or care, to my eyes, and I was a potential meal to him. I didn't see much else there.

He swam towards me steadily, swishing slightly back and forth, straight at me. Everything stopped inside of me. Everything anyone had ever said about what to do in this situation passed before my eyes and I knew it was all bullshit. There was nothing to do but to get out of the water. But I had to wait to see what he was going to do, what his move would be. He kept coming straight towards me, and my lungs began to ache. I couldn't hold on much longer, so just as he got to me, his big nose a foot in front of me, I kicked off, exploded from the ball I had been, and headed up toward a bright surface. I looked down the length of him, his nose inches away from my stomach. I twisted in the water, turned my back toward him and kicked for the surface.

Then everything became very quiet. I felt him behind me, below me, all around me, his eyes seeing me, his nose smelling me, his presence engulfing me. I left my body behind with him, from the waist down. In a moment that was like moving gelatin, I became only aware of my heart, my upper stomach, and my mind. All was very clear in these parts, while everything below that took on another dimension, one ready to transfer into another manner of being. Perhaps it would have been bloody, a sudden swirl of my blood and innards thrashing in the water silently. But it did not register to me. I had left home, and the presence in my upper body was colored by the cleanliness of what existed beyond even that, and that was a watery crisp knowing about something else beyond being even half a body. I prepared for death, while doing everything to escape it. It was the sudden calm mixed with panic, or fed by panic, the adrenaline truth of the spirit one has when a gun's cold muzzle touches his forehead. You know peace must be found very quickly.

Well, he didn't eat me, and I flew out of the water, landing in the middle of the boat without touching its sides. I smoked an unfiltered Camel down into a tiny nub, and still I shook all over. But even with all the shaking, I maintained a certain cool. I didn't yell for the joy of still living. I was gone, resting in some weird knowledge that it might have been better on the other side, or at least more tolerable and familiar.

So, when I went back to my meditation, I found that I had established a road for exit, and the process became easy from then on, yet I wanted more and more to live inside myself. At least so I thought, so I told myself. But I still courted the exit, and sought to see things from the outside, seeking the esoteric ability to observe from the top of the pine tree all the particulars of my life. To be, as Christ advertised, "In the world, but not of it."

I was still scared. But of what? Of living? Definitely. I didn't know what I was going to do in the face of many things, including people's awesome capability for cruelty and all-around stupidity. It was a dangerous world I lived in. In addition, I was equally afraid of dying, though I knew intuitively that I could handle it better than I could living at the time. There were fewer choices, and perhaps that in itself was the temptation to leave. How can you be wrong when you are moving into the next world? Adrenaline and abject horror had combined to show me how easy things might be.

Later, I read all the sutras, watching from the beach as our cooks dropped hand grenades into the bay to fetch our evening meals, fish floating to the surface dead. It all seemed incredibly primitive, and it still does. A few months later, I chose not to kill people, when presented with the opportunity. There really was no choice for me, but I had thought there was, because I had been trained to kill, and I knew hunting as a child.

So I kept looking to expand my meditation. The shark stayed with me as he is today, a brilliant and harsh grandfather reminding me of mortality each time I check into his emblazoned presence in my being. He's a friend now, but I still wouldn't trust him with my body.

What does all this mean to me now? In my memory I see a monk with a curled brow and brown robes sitting outside a temple on a hot day. There is a pain on the edges of his eyes, and he squints toward the sun. I approach him and sit silently for awhile, then ask him what he's contemplating. He tells me he seeks to leave his body, so I ask him why. He stares at me for a second and we both smile, then he says, "because it's fucking scary here." I laugh hard, then look closely at the moss on the old stone steps where we sit, fingering it soberly. When I look back at him he is crying, seemingly not from sadness, but from frustration. He doesn't know where to go. He shrugs angrily, raising his palms skyward, and I stare at his face, our eyes meeting. Later we drink a few beers and he tells me about the difference between celibacy and abstinence. He says that celibacy is a crime against nature, while abstinence is a matter of choice, and benefits the body and soul at once. I don't know much about this, but remember a year in my life without sex, and what that gave me.

When my old heater crackles in the middle of a cold night, it speaks in rhythms of three, made of predictable living steel. The heat comes and goes while it sings its song. All these ruminations fit into each other, the shark into the monk, the ancient steps into the heat of the sun. I could die tomorrow, and would be immensely sorry for all the life I could have lived, because things have changed for me. I am no longer afraid of living, but deeply caught within its marvel. At the same time, the fact that one part of me has stepped outside, makes death less fearsome, though I realize the academic nature of this notion. I am really equally afraid of everything, I tell myself, in a state where almost nothing surprises me, and everything lays me bare.

It's just that fear has taught me the value of what I live, is all I wanted to say, and this principle may extend through all the living churches we might see. The shark did not wear a priest's collar, though I can picture it on him right now, and the monk's smile did not contain a double row of dripping teeth. But they are interchangeable, and the manner of their swim through my mind and memory has a purpose beyond their specific shapes and times. They are each other, when it comes to how I live my life, when it comes to how I react to violence, or to argument, or to someone standing in my face. I don't want to die, in any form, but to live forever in the most sublime way possible. I don't want to argue about who's going to do the dishes or clean the toilet. I just want to do them. I see myself in heaven, beyond the pearly gates, leaning over with a dust pan and broom, sweeping heavenly dirt out of God's living room, scrubbing the toilet.

Now my face squints up at the ever-present sun and I think of the monk crying on the steps of Burma. I think there is much for him to cry about in this world, and much cleaning to be done while I am still alive.

## For The Manner of
## Our Continuation

*As each day compiles the future, it is my wish that our warmth may continue to deepen, that the touch of the surface may fall clearly into the center. To continue to gently fill is my desire, to fill to spilling over into the world around us quietly. I do not wish to stop, or to take a path aside from this soft strength, but to awaken into it each morning, with great care and ease. And when times are hard, as the world must bring trials, it is my wish that we hold firm together, trading strength, trading courage, trading into the meeting between our eyes. May we find what we need in this touch always, and may our circle roll through the sky a thousand years.*